+RC568 .C6 T72 1988

5 0664 01004313 3

RC
568
C6
T72
1988

Treating cocaine
dependency

DATE DUE

DEC 04 1993

NOV 02 1993

NOV 09 1995

AUDREY COHEN COLLEGE LIBRARY
345 HUDSON STREET
NEW YORK, NY 10014

Treating Cocaine Dependency

David E. Smith, M.D.
Donald R. Wesson, M.D.

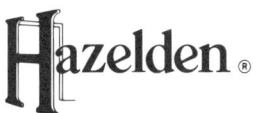

First published July, 1985.
Expanded edition published October, 1988.

Copyright © 1988, Hazelden Foundation.
All rights reserved. No portion of this publication
may be reproduced in any manner without the written
permission of the publisher.

ISBN: 0-89486-279-0

Printed in the United States of America.

Editor's Note:
 Hazelden Educational Materials offers a variety of information on chemical dependency and related areas. Our publications do not necessarily represent Hazelden or its programs, nor do they officially speak for any Twelve Step organization.
 Treating Cocaine Dependency was originally published as *Treating the Cocaine Abuser* by Hazelden Educational Materials.

About the book:
Cocaine use has reached epidemic proportions in the United States, raising questions about the drug's effects and approaches to treating the cocaine addict. This book provides an overview of crack and cocaine use, the medical effects of the drug, an analysis of addictive disease, information on treatment for codependents, and a description of cocaine-specific recovery groups.

About the authors:
David E. Smith, M.D., is the founder and Medical Director of the Haight-Ashbury Free Medical Clinic, Research Director at the Merritt Peralta Chemical Dependency Recovery Hospital, and Associate Clinical Professor in Toxicology at the University of California, San Francisco Medical Center.

Donald R. Wesson, M.D., is Assistant Clinical Professor, Department of Psychiatry, at the University of California, San Francisco, and at San Francisco Veterans Administration Medical Center, and is Science Director at the Merritt Peralta Chemical Dependency Recovery Hospital.

Joseph C. McCarthy, M.D., is the Medical Director of the John C. Lincoln Hospital Chemical Dependency Unit, and cofounder of the Cocaine Recovery Support Group, a research project of the Haight-Ashbury Free Medical Clinic.

Charles E. Nelson, Ph.D., is a psychotherapist in San Diego, and has specialized in treating cocaine abusers and codependents since 1976. He is an international consultant and trainer for chemical dependency treatment facilities.

Paul Ehrlich, M.A., is Program Director of Forest Farm, a residential chemical dependency program for adolescents and young adults. He is cofounder of the Cocaine Treatment and Research Project, a joint project between Forest Farm and the Haight-Ashbury Free Medical Clinic.

Maureen McGeehan, M.S.W., A.C.S.W., is a therapist in private practice and is working in the field of chemical dependency treatment.

Mim Landry is Director of the Training and Education Project at the Haight-Ashbury Free Medical Clinic in San Francisco.

CONTENTS

Chapter

	Introduction David E. Smith, M.D., and Donald R. Wesson, M.D.	1
1	Cocaine Abuse and Treatment: An Overview David E. Smith, M.D., and Donald R. Wesson, M.D.	5
2	The Concept of Addictive Disease Joseph C. McCarthy, M.D.	21
3	The Medical Complications of Cocaine Abuse Joseph C. McCarthy, M.D.	31
4	The Styles of Enabling Behavior Charles E. Nelson, Ph.D.	49
5	Cocaine Recovery Support Groups: The Language of Recovery Paul Ehrlich, M.A. Maureen McGeehan, M.S.W., A.C.S.W.	73
	Appendix Update on Cocaine Dependence: Crack and Advances in Diagnostics and Treatment Mim Landry	91

INTRODUCTION

Cocaine is a powerful central nervous system stimulant that has received great public and media attention in recent years. An estimated 24 million Americans have tried cocaine, and two to four million use it on a regular basis. The cost of cocaine use in the United States has fueled a multibillion dollar illicit industry. Despite strict laws prohibiting cocaine use and intense law enforcement efforts aimed at cocaine smugglers, primarily in Central and South America where the coca plant is grown, many of our major urban areas are glutted with cocaine with the purity of the drug increasing and the price decreasing.

With wider acceptance of cocaine use in the United States, changing rituals and patterns of use, and usage methods resulting in a more rapid intoxication (such as smoking cocaine freebase), health problems have also increased. There is a substantial increase in cocaine overdose cases coming into emergency rooms and drug treatment programs, a major increase in people with medical and psychiatric complications of cocaine abuse seeking attention in the health care system, and a growing number of people who realize their use is out of control seeking help in long-term chemical dependency programs.

This book provides a multidisciplinary epidemiological, diagnostic, and treatment perspective on current patterns of cocaine abuse in the United States. It describes patterns of cocaine abuse and the basic pharmacology of the drug.

Treatment of medical and psychiatric complications are outlined, and long-term treatment strategies for recovery from cocaine addiction are emphasized.

Many characteristics of the epidemic of cocaine abuse are new, but based on our twenty years of experience in studying cocaine, it is apparent much of what we have learned in the developing field of chemical dependency, particularly in the area of alcoholism, is applicable to the diagnosis and treatment of cocaine addiction. Addictive disease is a pathological process with characteristic signs and symptoms and a predictable prognosis. If untreated, it is a progressive and potentially fatal illness, and it is obvious that a subgroup of our population exposed to cocaine will develop addictive disease. It is important that the disease concept as outlined in this book be understood by the treatment team as well as the individual afflicted with the problem of chemical dependency.

Cocaine addiction is a multifaceted disease with physical, psychological, pharmacological, behavioral, and spiritual components. The complications vary in severity depending on the progression of the disease. With this in mind, a continuum of care must be emphasized, including inpatient chemical dependency treatment, long-term residential care, outpatient treatment, and recovery groups compatible with the Twelve Steps of recovery originally outlined by Alcoholics Anonymous, the grandfather of all recovery groups. Since a majority of cocaine abusers also abuse other drugs, particularly depressants such as alcohol, prescription sedative-hypnotics, or narcotics in an upper-downer cycle, clinicians treating addiction must be familiar with cross-addiction theory. In the long-term, the cocaine addict does best if he or she evolves toward a chemical-free philosophy that emphasizes abstinence from all major mood-altering drugs and is coupled with participation in an ongoing recovery group process. It is also clear that the expanding work with families of chemically dependent patients, best developed in the field of alcoholism, is also applicable to the problem of cocaine addiction. Toward this end, it is important to emphasize family education and treatment.

This book is intended for a multidisciplinary team, although specific chapters may be more applicable to the work of a particular discipline. We hope, however, that readers will look at all chapters in this book, rather than just the ones applicable to their own discipline. For example, physicians treating the complications of cocaine addiction may find the chapters on overdose and detoxification management are most appropriate for their work. However, management of the complications of the disease are not synonymous with the management of the disease itself, where much of the long-term approach is nonmedical in nature. To understand this nonmedical, long-term treatment approach, physicians should become familiar with the group process and understand the language of recovery. Conversely, clinicians working primarily with long-term recovery issues or family therapy programs should have a basic understanding of the medical chapters to improve their educational and diagnostic skills. We hope this multidisciplinary book can serve all members of the treatment team, since clearly effective treatment of chemical dependency requires a health care team approach, involving both professional and nonprofessional members as well as recovering and nonrecovering members. Each member of the chemical dependency treatment team should have some awareness of the other's role in order to provide more effective treatment for the individual with addictive disease. All members of the team should be clear in their perception of the addictive process in order to more effectively communicate with other members of the team.

This book assumes cocaine addiction is a progressive and potentially fatal disease with great potential for relapse, particularly if the individual attempts a return to controlled use of the drug. It also assumes, however, that this disease is a treatable illness. With effective treatment, the fatal course can be altered and those affected can live a comfortable and responsible life without the use of psychoactive drugs, thus saving themselves, their families, and society the many complications of addictive disease. We hope the readers of this book will both share and refine these assumptions into beliefs as we attempt to deal effectively with the cocaine abuse epidemic in the United States.

David E. Smith, M.D., and Donald R. Wesson, M.D.
March, 1985

1
COCAINE ABUSE AND TREATMENT: AN OVERVIEW

David E. Smith, M.D.
Donald R. Wesson, M.D.

USE AND ABUSE

Before the mid-1960s, when cocaine use was primarily by heroin addicts and other members of the hard-core drug culture, the majority of Americans regarded cocaine users as criminals. Cocaine had little appeal for those not associated with socially deviant behavior.

During the late 1960s and early 1970s, many people changed their attitudes about cocaine, and subsequently cocaine began to be used by a broad segment of American society. The attitude shift preceded widespread use and occurred for many reasons. Important among them was a liberalization of attitudes about recreational drug use caused by the wider acceptance of marijuana use. Cocaine use became viewed as analogous to marijuana use; both were illegal, but their use was not viewed by most Americans as criminal behavior. With marijuana this attitude was reflected in laws which decriminalized possession for personal use, but escalated penalties for marijuana sellers.

The media, by allocating a disproportionate amount of attention to cocaine, played a significant role in its popularization. By treating the lifestyle of affluent upper-class drug dealers and the use of cocaine by celebrities as newsworthy, the mass media in essence created an advertising campaign for cocaine, and many people were encouraged to perceive cocaine as chic, exclusive, daring, and nonaddicting. Television specials about cocaine abuse showed scientists describing the extraordinary feats laboratory animals would perform to receive cocaine injections. Likewise, clinicians who treated drug dependency contributed to cocaine's mystique by reporting case histories of patients who became so preoccupied with using cocaine they lost their families, jobs, and careers. Since people don't really believe they will become "victims" (the same denial mechanism that allows people to smoke cigarettes), the addictive potential of cocaine is more of an enticement to use it, rather than a deterrent.

The portrayal of cocaine as dangerous may even add appeal for the adventuresome. Consider, for example, the message conveyed by the March, 1985 cover of *Discovery Magazine*. A pile of white crystalline powder, two lines of powder, and a single edged razor blade are shown on a blue background. Below them in bold yellow letters is the following text:

> This amount of cocaine can make you feel that you're brilliant, tireless, masterful, invulnerable, and that you're going to live forever. It can also kill you.

The cost of cocaine is kept high by demand and interdiction of supply by law enforcement. Although keeping the price high by limiting supplies limits the amount of cocaine accessible to some users and is a deterrent to some experimental use and socio-recreational use, especially by youth, the high price also reinforces its elite status.

The decline in amphetamine availability may also have been a factor favoring cocaine's popularity. In the mid-1970s, many drug users were using stimulants. Amphetamine, which previously had been readily available from physicians' prescriptions or from diversion of pharmaceutically manufactured supplies, became difficult for most people to acquire. After amphetamines were moved to Schedule II, physicians were reluctant to prescribe them, and the amount available from diversion of pharmaceutically manufactured amphetamines declined. This decrease was due in great part to effective regulation of legitimate amphetamine production and distribution. At the same time, the black market was glutted by amphetamine look-alikes which contained ephedrine, phenylpropanolamine, and caffeine.

Still another factor which favored the popularization of cocaine was professional and lay misunderstanding of the relationship between physical dependence and addiction. Models of addiction have morphine or heroin as the prototype, and addiction was assumed to require both tolerance and physical dependence. Since cocaine has no obvious withdrawal syndrome in animals, many people believe cocaine is not addicting. Part of the confusion has been semantic because the term *addiction* has so many different meanings. But the notion that cocaine was not addicting because it did not induce physical dependence was important in the initial popularization of cocaine. It is less important today as fewer people still believe that cocaine is nonaddicting.

With cocaine's increasing social acceptance, the number of users has increased among a diverse group of people — from professionals to street heroin addicts. A national household survey of drug use conducted in 1982 showed that 28 percent of young adults 18 to 25 years of age had used cocaine on one or more occasions.[1] The relationship of the number of people who have ever used cocaine to prevalence of cocaine abuse is not known with precision, however, it is certainly a measure of public acceptance and popularity.

Other notions about the prevalence of cocaine use are derived from drug treatment experiences. Cocaine is increasingly given as the primary drug of abuse by people seeking treatment for drug addiction in both the public and private treatment sectors. However, part of the increase is misleading as polydrug abusers will claim cocaine dependency — even though it is not their primary drug of abuse — because cocaine is fashionable. But while some distortion of cocaine treatment statistics is produced by overacclaim, increases in the number of problems associated with cocaine abuse are real. Cocaine abuse is more conspicuous to private physicians because growing numbers of people are seeking treatment for complications of cocaine abuse: toxic psychosis, overdose, addiction, and even for a previously rare problem — a perforated nasal septum.

Proprietary drug treatment programs have responded resourcefully to the cocaine casualties of the affluent and medically insured, and they have devised treatment modalities specifically tailored to cocaine abuse: cocaine recovery support groups, resort retreats, aversive therapy, and short and long-term residential treatment.

Although more people are coming to treatment for cocaine abuse (as well as attending cocaine recovery support groups and Cocaine Anonymous), the rising number of people requesting treatment does not necessarily reflect increasing prevalence of cocaine use in the total population. Some people use cocaine for several years before they develop dependency or medical complications, and many users experiment with cocaine and never require treatment. Many cocaine abusers now seeking treatment are multiple drug abusers with cocaine being the pivotal drug bringing them to treatment.

In spite of the availability of private, hospital-based treatment programs, growing numbers of middle- and upper-class people are seeking treatment for their cocaine abuse problems in alternative care facilities such as the Haight-Ashbury Free Medical Clinic. This occurs for several reasons. Many cocaine abusers who are still working seek help in alternative care clinics where medical insurance billing, often handled by their employers, will not be involved. They are concerned that the insurance diagnosis would inform their employer of their cocaine abuse. For the same reason, many cocaine abusers will not seek treatment with their private physician or in a public drug treatment facility.

COCAINE AVAILABILITY

Deception is the rule in the illicit drug marketplace. Cocaine may be cut with lidocaine, tetracaine, mannitol, caffeine, or amphetamine, and the actual amount of cocaine in street samples varies widely. When treating a cocaine overdose, the toxicity of contaminants, "cuts," and substitutes must be considered.

Until recently, cocaine hydrochloride, the water-soluble salt, was the usual form of cocaine sold. Users who wanted cocaine freebase had to make their own from cocaine hydrochloride. Freebase kits containing the necessary reagents (a strong base such as sodium hydroxide and an organic solvent such as ether) were available for mail-order purchase or were sold in drug paraphernalia shops. The freebase kits have been removed from legitimate purchase in some states. Freebase use continues, however, as some methods of making freebase do not need the reagents and because cocaine is now sometimes sold in freebase form. On the west coast of the U.S., cocaine freebase is sold under the name of "rock." Cocaine freebase crystals are compacted into a "rock" which can be broken up and smoked without further preparation. Rock cocaine is sold from "rock houses" which may also provide a place to smoke cocaine freebase and use other drugs such as heroin to manage anxiety reactions, irritability, and paranoia.

Cocaine Use by Health Professionals

Since cocaine is available for medicinal uses through pharmaceutical suppliers, one might suppose that physicians who use cocaine for recreational purposes would acquire their supply from pharmaceutical sources. Except for ear, nose, and throat specialists and anesthesiologists, most physicians acquire cocaine for their personal use through the illicit marketplace because they are concerned that ordering cocaine would invite discovery of their drug use. Hospital pharmacists who work where large amounts of cocaine are used for surgery or for preparation of Brompton's solution (an oral pain-relieving medication for terminal cancer patients containing a narcotic — usually methadone or morphine — cocaine, and alcohol) have access to pharmaceutical cocaine.

Cocaine Look-alikes

Drug paraphernalia businesses are attempting to capitalize on cocaine's popularity by offering for sale uncontrolled substances simulating the properties of cocaine (sold under names such as Peruvian Flake, Snocaine, and Hard Rock Crystal). These products are nationally advertised for mail-order purchase in sexually explicit magazines and are also sold in drug paraphernalia shops. They may contain, alone or in combination, lidocaine, tetracaine, caffeine, or phenylpropanolamine. They are sold as incense and labeled with a disclaimer, "not for drug use," in an effort to elude regulations applicable to drugs.

DIAGNOSIS OF COCAINE ABUSE

Using the social diagnosis of drug abuse — i.e., the "use, usually by self-administration, of any drug in a manner that deviates from the approved medical or social patterns within a given culture"[2] — any use of cocaine would be considered abuse. A clinician, however, needs a diagnosis which makes a distinction between *cocaine use* which, although not socially sanctioned, is experimental or noncompulsive socio-recreational use and *cocaine abuse* which requires treatment. The diagnosis of cocaine abuse used by many clinicians and most researchers is that of the Third Edition of the American Psychiatric Association's *Diagnostic and Statistical Manual of Mental Disorders (DSM III).*[3] The *DSM III* criteria do not equate use and abuse as would the social definition of cocaine abuse. Cocaine abuse requires a pattern of *pathological use:*

inability to reduce or stop use, intoxication throughout the day, and episodes of cocaine overdose, impairment of social or occupational functioning, and a duration of disturbance for more than one month.

The issue of physical dependence on cocaine is still controversial — especially among animal pharmacologists. The *DSM III* reflects this controversy by not including a diagnostic category for cocaine dependence (only a category of cocaine abuse is included). A diagnostic category of cocaine dependence is not given in *DSM III* because "the withdrawal symptoms are transitory." This is a *non sequitur* as withdrawal symptoms from heroin are also transitory. Experienced clinicians attribute two types of reactions to withdrawal: (1) following a short, high-dose binge of cocaine use, there is a two to four day period in which the person is apathetically depressed, fatigued, and exhausted; (2) following chronic high doses of cocaine, the withdrawal period is characterized by dysphoria, lethargy, insomnia, and irritability.

Addiction

We define addiction as compulsion to use a drug, loss of control over the amount used, and continued use in spite of adverse consequences. Using this definition, cocaine is unquestionably addicting. The cocaine patients we have treated used cocaine compulsively and their use was limited only by cocaine availability or legal, medical, or psychiatric complications. They continued to use despite loss of their personal or business financial resources, the negative impact on their marriages and families, and deterioration of their work capacity or employment. Even within the structure of an outpatient recovery program, many cocaine abusers have great difficulty remaining cocaine-free.

Use of Drug Combinations

Few cocaine abusers use only cocaine. Cocaine abusers often use barbiturates, methaqualone, benzodiazepines, or alcohol to self-medicate insomnia, agitation, and irritability which result from their cocaine use. Thus they develop an upper-downer syndrome similar to that associated with amphetamine use.[4] The simultaneous use of intoxicating amounts of stimulants and sedative-hypnotics can produce disastrous consequences. The intoxicated person has the gross impairment of judgment and motor skills produced by the sedative-hypnotic and the energy to remain awake and active due to the stimulant.

The use of alcohol or other depressants to relieve cocaine's side effects may result in a secondary dependence on sedatives. People with combined alcohol dependence and cocaine abuse often seek treatment in alcohol treatment centers. Many then encounter inadequate information about treatment of cocaine abuse and ambivalent attitudes toward treatment of mixed drug and alcohol addiction.

Instead of, or in addition to, sedatives, some high-dose cocaine abusers may also try to medicate the side effects of cocaine with opiates such as heroin, meperidine (Demerol), or other prescription opiates. Dual physical dependence on cocaine and alcohol, or cocaine and opiates complicates withdrawal and increases the severity of the withdrawal syndrome.

Cocaine Freebase

Smoking cocaine freebase in the United States was predated by the smoking of coca paste in Peru.[5] Cocaine freebase use is associated in the San Francisco Bay Area with a parallel increase in the smoking of Persian heroin.[6] Cocaine users may begin smoking Persian heroin to reduce the agitation produced by cocaine. After using heroin several times, they may then acquire a desire for heroin and become primary heroin abusers or mixed heroin and cocaine abusers. Many freebase users are middle-class, have no previous experience with the drug treatment system and have short addiction histories. Because many of these people believe that "if you don't stick a needle in your arm, you can't be an addict," denial of addiction is a common obstacle to treatment. Contrary to their belief, smoking Persian heroin produces physical dependence of the opiate type, and opiate withdrawal symptoms will occur when use is abruptly stopped. Thus, despite their denial of addiction and unusual demographic profile, these users often arrive for treatment with physical dependence on opiates.

Intravenous Injection of Cocaine

Cocaine hydrochloride can be dissolved in water and injected. Some cocaine abusers realize that the injection is a more efficient means of using cocaine and convert from snorting or freebasing to injecting cocaine. For these users, cocaine may be the first drug injected. Usually, however, intravenous cocaine abusers come from the ranks of intravenous heroin users who already know the injection mode.

Some abusers combine heroin and cocaine. The combination, known as a speedball, has been familiar for many years to hard-core drug users who inject the mixture. Some users now smoke a combination of cocaine freebase and Persian heroin. We have treated patients who developed opiate dependency using this combination. When Persian heroin decreased in availability or quality, some users began using heroin intravenously because injection is more efficient than smoking.

COMPLICATIONS OF COCAINE USE

When a society first incorporates a new, powerful intoxicant high morbidity always occurs; therefore abuse, morbidity, and mortality are expected. Cocaine, alone and in combination with other drugs, is responsible for many serious medical and psychiatric complications. When cocaine is injected intravenously, many complications occur which are common to illicit needle use such as abscesses and injection of bacteria and particulate matter. But whether used by injection, smoking, or inhalation, some complications of cocaine are the result of its specific pharmacology.

The medical complications of cocaine are covered in detail in Chapter 3. Some of the more common medical complications and psychological consequences will be discussed here.

Adverse Cardiac Effects

The cardiac consequences of cocaine use include tachycardia, hypertension, and ventricular arrythmias. In some instances, the cardiac effects can be fatal. For example, a case of myocardial infarction has been reported in a 38-year-old male associated with snorting cocaine.[7]

Seizures

An overdose of cocaine can cause grand mal seizures. Intravenous diazepam and support of the cardio-respiratory system for status epilepticus or post-seizure depression are the appropriate techniques for management of the cocaine-induced seizure.

Death

In most fatal cocaine overdoses, the mechanism of death appears to be respiratory arrest or cardiac arrythmia. Although most fatalities occur among those who have injected cocaine or smoked it in its freebase form, deaths also occur with cocaine snorting. Deaths from body packing (smugglers concealing the drug in their stomach or intestinal tracts) also have occurred when the storage containers burst and the smuggler's body received a massive amount of cocaine.[8]

Psychological Complications

Cocaine can produce a broad range of psychological effects, ranging from acute anxiety to full-blown cocaine psychosis with paranoia and auditory and visual hallucinations. These toxic reactions are dose related and depend on physical tolerance to the drug, psychological set, and socio-cultural setting. Acute anxiety reaction or the "overamp" dysphoria described by the cocaine abusers usually can be managed in an outpatient setting with reassurance, a supportive environment, and oral sedative-hypnotic medications such as diazepam.

As with amphetamine, prolonged high-dose administration of cocaine in the one to four grams a day dosage range is associated with sleep deprivation and cocaine psychosis — auditory and visual hallucinations and paranoia with ideas of reference. We have seen a substantial increase in cocaine psychosis at the Haight-Ashbury Free Medical Clinic due to abuse of cocaine freebase.

Qualitatively, the cocaine psychosis is similar to the amphetamine psychosis but shorter in duration. With a structured outpatient setting, we have been able to manage these cocaine psychoses with the use of two mg of haloperidol (Haldol) every four hours. If this amount of haloperidol does not control paranoia and other acute psychotic symptoms, psychiatric hospitalization and higher dosages of haloperidol are indicated.

Combined Psychiatric Disorders and Cocaine Abuse

Occasionally individuals with underlying thought disorders have a more prolonged psychotic reaction that is precipitated by cocaine. They often have a family history of schizophrenia, and the prolonged psychosis probably is a cocaine-precipitated schizophrenic reaction. These cases are also frequently complicated by multiple drug abuse.

Sexual Dysfunction

Cocaine affects sexual functioning in ways similar to amphetamine. At low doses, cocaine enhances sexual desire and is highly rated as an aphrodisiac in the drug culture, especially by males. However, as the dosage increases and use becomes chronic, particularly if the route of administration is freebase smoking or injection, a male's ejaculatory and erectile ability may be impaired, and women may find difficulty having orgasm. In a study of cocaine use in massage parlors, masseuses reported males valued cocaine because of delayed ejaculation, but often erectile performance was so impaired that erection would not occur.[9] Certainly chronic, high-dose cocaine abuse can induce severe sexual dysfunction and this is one reason users seek treatment. For that reason, awareness of sexual dysfunction is important for treatment personnel.[10]

High doses of cocaine, like high doses of amphetamine, also can facilitate sexual behavior such as compulsive masturbation or multipartner marathons that the individual self-defines as aberrant and unhealthy.

✓TREATMENT OF COCAINE DEPENDENCE

Many cocaine abusers enter treatment with the hope of learning controlled use of cocaine. Others may accept the need to relinquish all cocaine use, but they do not see the need to relinquish use of alcohol or other psychotropic drugs which have not resulted in addictive behavior. However, once a person has become an abuser of cocaine the most efficacious treatment is complete abstinence from all psychotropic drugs.

There are many reasons to recommend total abstinence. First, use of any drug of abuse alienates the person from recovery-oriented group support. Second, use of a drug such as alcohol, even if not previously a drug of abuse for the person, is unwise because while under the influence of the alcohol, the person's resolve to avoid cocaine use is lessened. Third, a person who seeks to alter consciousness by using one drug may well substitute another when the preferred drug is unavailable (i.e., cross-addiction).

Withdrawal

As previously mentioned, physical dependence on cocaine is controversial; however, the withdrawal period for chronic abusers is characterized by a sad mood, agitation, lethargy, insomnia, and irritability. This cluster of symptoms appears to respond, in uncontrolled studies, to L-tryptophan, the amino acid precursor to serotonin, in dosages of 2000 mg to 6000 mg per day. This dose appears effective in reducing anxiety, agitation, and insomnia associated with stimulant withdrawal. We do not employ tricyclic antidepressants for cocaine withdrawal depression unless there is clear evidence for a depressive disorder unrelated to cocaine use.

Relapse

Relapse to cocaine abuse usually occurs in stages. First, the person decides that he or she is finally "cured" and can therefore drop therapy, group support, or drug treatment aftercare. A common second step is to experiment with some drug other than cocaine (e.g., alcohol or marijuana) and find that loss of control or relapse to cocaine abuse does not occur. Next, the person may use a small amount of cocaine and when immediate loss of control does not occur, the person is convinced that a cure has occurred and that episodic, careful use of cocaine is reasonable. Finally, with repeated episodes of cocaine use, loss of control eventually recurs, and the relapse is complete. Thus, once a person has lost the ability to control the amount of a drug used except by availability, the person should maintain complete abstinence from all drugs of abuse and never attempt to return to controlled use of drugs.

Recovery

For most cocaine abusers, the focus of treatment needs to be on the toxic consequences of cocaine, with cocaine-free recovery as the goal. This is best accomplished through a combination of individual and group therapy provided in an outpatient setting. Initial treatment may need to be inpatient if the patient is unable to secure a sustained period of abstinence or if cocaine toxicity has impaired judgement. Principles of recovery and constructive alternatives as a way of dealing with cocaine hunger are stressed. A positive approach to recovery, in contrast to "white knuckle sobriety," is fostered. The recovery process requires substantial education of the client on addictive disease generally and on cocaine abuse specifically. Including family members in the recovery process increases the chances of success, and in most cases recovery is enhanced by family therapy.

Group therapy is a vital component of the recovery program. In cocaine recovery groups, discussed in detail by Paul Ehrlich and Maureen McGeehan in Chapter Five, recovering cocaine abusers support one another in their efforts to cope with cocaine hunger. Having the groups composed of patients who are in different stages of recovery is helpful. Patients with a short period of recovery often do not *really believe* long-term abstinence is possible. Having people with long periods of abstinence in the group reinforces the possibility of recovery and supports the positive aspects of giving up drug use. Such patients with long-term recovery can also add support to the notion that cocaine cravings become less intense and less frequent the longer one is abstinent.

Cocaine Anonymous groups, modelled after Alcoholics Anonymous and Narcotics Anonymous, are now available in some areas and are a valuable resource for recovering cocaine abusers. A.A. and N.A. also are useful to cocaine abusers in maintaining recovery. Since cocaine abusers may abuse other drugs, particularly alcohol, during the recovery phase, participation in these groups may be especially desirable.

Exercise as an Adjunct to Recovery

Other important aspects of recovery may include an exercise program where the individual uses the exercise not only to improve general health, but also to combat drug hunger. Exercise that produces cardiopulmonary stimulation for more than twenty minutes can produce an increase in the release of endorphins, followed by a reduction in drug hunger and anxiety. We regularly use the exercise alternative as part of the cocaine recovery program to reduce drug hunger and enhance self-image.

SUMMARY

Recovery from cocaine abuse is more than abstinence from cocaine, it is the pursuit of a different lifestyle. The term *cure* in the sense that the person can return to controlled cocaine use has no place in an effective recovery program. Attempts to return to controlled use must be defined as a slip or a relapse. During the recovery period, anticipatory guidance should be given to the client regarding the sequence of drug dreams, cocaine drug hunger, and addictive thinking that may predate a relapse. Silence is the enemy of recovery, and frequent open discussions supplemented with positive alternatives to using cocaine are necessary to interrupt this sequence and thereby prevent relapse. Instead, it is important to stress that recovery — meaning no psychoactive drug use and active participation in relapse prevention through peer support — is possible and can be a positive, life-enhancing process.

Chapter 1
ENDNOTES

1. J. D. Miller et al. *National Survey on Drug Abuse: Main Findings 1982.* National Institute on Drug Abuse. DHHS Pub. No. (ADM)83-1263. (Washington, D.C.: Supt. of Docs., U.S. Govt. Print. Off., 1983.)

2. J. H. Jaffe, "Drug Addiction and Drug Abuse," in *The Pharmacological Basis of Therapeutics,* sixth edition, A. G. Gilman, L. S. Goodman, and A. Gilman, eds., (New York: MacMillan Publishing Co., 1980), p. 535.
3. American Psychiatric Association. *Diagnostic and Statistical Manual of Mental Disorders (DSM III),* third edition, (Washington, D.C.: American Psychiatric Association, 1980)
4. D. E. Smith and D. R. Wesson, *Uppers and Downers.* (Englewood Cliffs, New Jersey: Prentice-Hall, Inc., 1973)
5. F. R. Jeri, C. Sanchez, T. del Dozo, "The Syndrome of Coca Paste: Observations in a Group of Patients in the Lima Area." *Journal of Psychoactive Drugs,* Volume 10, (1978) pp.361-370.
6. D. E. Smith et al. "Persian Heroin in the San Francisco Bay Area, 1977-1980: The New Wave?" *California Society for the Treatment of Alcoholism and Other Drug Dependencies Newsletter.* Volume 7 April, 1980.
7. D. L. Coleman, T. Ross, and J. Naughton, "Myocardial Ischemia and Infarction Related to Recreational Cocaine Use." *Western Journal of Medicine,* Volume 136, 1982, pp. 444-446.
8. C. V. Wetli and R. E. Mittleman, "The 'Body Packer Syndrome': Toxicity Following Ingestion of Illicit Drugs Packaged for Transportation." *Journal of Forensic Science,* Volume 26, (1981), p. 492.
9. D. R. Wesson, "Cocaine Use by Masseuses," *Journal of Psychoactive Drugs,* Volume 14, (1982) pp. 75-76.
10. D. E. Smith, D. R. Wesson, and M. Apter-Marsh, "Cocaine and Alcohol-induced Sexual Dysfunction in Patients with Addictive Disease," *Journal of Psychoactive Drugs,* Volume 16, (1984) pp. 359-360.

2
THE CONCEPT OF ADDICTIVE DISEASE
Joseph C. McCarthy, M.D.

ADDICTION AS DISEASE

The treatment of chemical dependency has undergone dramatic changes during the past several years. One of the factors which has stimulated this change is the increasing acceptance of addiction as a disease. Since Jellinek first proposed this concept in 1960[1] with specific reference to alcohol, it has been broadened to include all psychoactive drugs. However, misunderstanding and controversy in this area still exist. This paper will present an updated and expanded statement of this concept with particular reference to cocaine.

In examining addictive disease, it is useful to define the terms. *Addictive* comes from the Latin *addictus,* which means "to devote or give oneself up habitually to something." A disease, on the other hand, is a definite morbid process having a characteristic train of symptoms; it may affect the whole body or any of its parts, and its etiology, pathology, and prognosis may be known or unknown."[2] In this case the "something" is a psychoactive drug, i.e., any drug which has an effect on the mind. So when we say a person has addictive disease we are saying this person is involved in an unhealthy process which affects the whole body and leads to a characteristic train of symptoms. The cause of this unhealthy process is the habitual use of a psychoactive drug, and the results of this use produce predictable adverse effects. These adverse effects may be physical, mental, social, or financial; and in most cases, all of these domains are affected. Furthermore, although the individual psychoactive drugs may produce different specific adverse effects, the basic underlying addictive process is the same.

Having defined addictive disease, how can one recognize those who have the disease? One way is by their behavioral characteristics.

1. *Compulsion.* Users with addictive disease manifest drug-seeking and drug-using behavior. When the drug is not present, the drive is to obtain the drug. When the drug is present, the drive is to use the drug and then the cycle repeats and reinforces itself. It is important to stress that this pattern may be episodic rather than continuous. The drug dictates behavior, and drug use temporarily satisfies drug hunger.

2. *Loss of control.* The issue of controlling one's drug use is limited to the person with addictive disease. Social drug users are not generally concerned with the issue of control. The addicted user may adopt many strategies in an attempt to control use. The alcoholic may attempt to drink only after 5 P.M. or only on weekends or may decide to drink only beer or wine. The cocaine user may buy only 1/4 gram at a time, and when this has been used he or she will buy an additional 1/4 gram; this pattern will continue until large quantities of the drug have been consumed. As the disease progresses, this loss of control becomes more frequent, and in the late stages of the disease the addiction is so powerful that drug use causes an addict to completely lose control.

3. *Continued use in spite of adverse consequences.* For the nonaddicted user, adverse consequences in the physical, mental, social, or financial sphere will usually curtail or modify drug use. With the addicted user, the same adverse consequences will often be ignored or denied until the situation becomes nearly catastrophic. Even at that point, some external event is required before a change in behavior takes place.

TYPES OF DRUG USE

Using these behavioral criteria, it is possible to separate those with addictive disease from those who are "recreational" drug users.

Under the heading of recreational users it is possible to classify three subtypes.

1. *Experimental.* This person has tried the drug once, or only a few times. Since the experience was neutral or even negative, he or she would not use the drug again. The experimental cocaine user, for example, may have snorted a few lines and found the drug did not produce the expected euphoria or even produced some dysphoria. After a second similar experience with the drug, he or she would not use the drug again.

2. *Occasional.* This is the "social" user who will indulge in drug use occasionally. This use occurs most often in a social setting such as a party. The use is low level, and the user does not experience any adverse consequences as a result. In the case of an occasional cocaine user, the quantity would rarely exceed 1/4 gram and the route of administration would be intranasal. Remember that most addicts were in this stage early in their using careers.

3. *Abuse.* This person may occasionally abuse the drug by becoming intoxicated. The cocaine user who falls into this category will use increasing quantities of the drug (1/2 -1 gram) and will frequently begin to experiment with intravenous drug injection or cocaine freebase smoking. This type of abuse is the result of a conscious, cognitive decision to abuse the drug and differs qualitatively from addictive use. The transition from a social user to an abuser is a difference in degree; the transition from an abuser to an addicted user is a difference in kind. The abuser may, for any number of reasons, choose to limit his or her drug use and revert to being a social user. However, given time, continued exposure

to the drug, and the proper biochemical/genetic predisposition, the abuser may progress to addictive use.

Progression is always from recreational use to addictive use. For some, this may involve a very short time frame and for others it may take years. Once addicted, no return to recreational use is possible. This is worth reemphasizing since every addict's fondest wish is to return to recreational use. Alcoholics Anonymous has a wonderful expression which graphically illustrates this concept. Recreational drug users are considered cucumbers, and addictive drug users are considered pickles. Under the right conditions a cucumber may become a pickle, but under no circumstances can a pickle ever return to being a cucumber.

BIOCHEMICAL/GENETIC DISORDER

I consider addictive disease to be primarily a biochemical/genetic disorder which is activated by the environment. The genetic predisposition to alcoholism has been well established by Goodwin and others.[3] While other psychoactive drugs have been less well studied, there does appear to be higher incidence of psychoactive drug addiction in the families of addicts than in the population at large. Millicent Buxton and Marty Jessup, R.N., of the Bay Area Task Force for Impaired Nurses, have noted that 65% of all meperidine (Demerol) addicts in the Bay Area Nurses Support Group have a positive family history of addiction.[4] Additional support for this viewpoint is provided by Smith, who states that 70% of all cocaine addicts have a family history of alcoholism.[5]

The evidence for cross-addiction, particularly among cocaine users, is strong. Gold reports that almost 70% of 500 randomly selected cocaine users who called the 800-COCAINE hot line used alcohol, heroin, or other narcotics in conjunction with their cocaine.[6]

A number of centers are engaged in animal research which

focuses specifically on the biochemical nature of addiction. While the research is preliminary, some exciting findings in the fields of endorphin/enkephalin physiology, tetrahydroisoquinolone formation and actions, and receptor site crossover effects of various classes of drugs are beginning to give us a foothold in this area. It is expected that further research in this area will yield specific biochemical differences between those with addictive disease and their nonaddicted counterparts.

OTHER CHARACTERISTICS OF ADDICTIVE DISEASE

While those with addictive disease can be separated from their peers by certain behavioral characteristics of their drug use, a number of additional characteristics of the disease itself are pertinent.

1. *Chronic.* Addictive disease is a chronic disease as opposed to an acute disease. As such, it is not curable, although it is amenable to treatment. Since continued exposure to the drug causes the disease to progress, treatment consists of abstinence and involvement in the process of recovery.

2. *Primary and simple.* Drug hunger and the desire to use are very basic drives in the addict. They often rise up with a primitive kind of energy and overpower all mental constraints, resolutions, and prohibitions. In addition, no other disease process is necessary for addictive disease to manifest itself. The individual may be in excellent health with the exception of the consequences of addictive drug use.

3. *Progressive.* The disease progresses over time and in its sensitivity to the drug. Thus the disease can be divided into early, middle, and late stages. The early stage is characterized by the use of increasing amounts of the drug and increasing tolerance to its effects. The middle stage is heralded by the presence of withdrawal symptoms and the onset of tissue toxicity and physical disease. The late stage is rapidly

progressive and presents with decreasing tolerance, physical and mental deterioration, and, if use continues, death.

4. *Predisposed to relapse.* Relapse occurs so frequently it should be considered an integral part of the disease. It is unusual for a person to get into recovery and never have a relapse. The relapse tends to escalate rapidly once it begins and impressive toxicity may occur, even with short periods of drug use. Unfortunately, any relapse may be fatal.

5. *Fatal.* Addictive disease is a potentially fatal disease. Because of the many complications associated with addictive drug use, premature death is not an unusual outcome. Since this is the case, the disease should be treated aggressively and with the same sense of urgency and commitment engendered by other potentially fatal diseases.

SUSCEPTIBILITY AND EXPOSURE

It is often difficult to explain why some people who use drugs never develop addictive disease, while others seemingly develop it with their first exposure. While future research may provide a definitive answer, some light can be shed on the problem by an examination of the role of susceptibility and exposure.

In the early part of the twentieth century, tuberculosis was a leading cause of death in the United States. At that time, some people were able to work with tubercular patients for years and yet they never contracted clinical tuberculosis. These people may be considered to have had a low susceptibility and would therefore only contract the disease after prolonged and intense exposure. On the other hand, other workers on the medical wards contracted the disease after only a brief exposure and died a short time later. They may be considered to have had high susceptibility and therefore required only a brief exposure. In the same way, those who use drugs for a long period of time and do not develop addictive disease may be considered to have a low susceptibility and insufficient exposure to develop clinical addictive disease. Conversely, those who use addictively almost from the beginning may have very high susceptibility and thus require only low exposure.

PSYCHOLOGY AND ADDICTION

My experience is that psychotherapy as a primary modality for the treatment of addictive disease is almost universally unsuccessful and potentially hazardous. The belief that addictive disease is due primarily to psychological factors is, unfortunately, still widely held. This system of belief holds that the basis for addictive drug use lies in the psychological makeup of the addicted person and that there is an *addictive personality*. The logical corollary of this view is that the primary treatment for addictive disease should be psychotherapy.

In his excellent prospective study of more than 600 patients over 40 years, Vaillant points out that "when other more salient variables like culture and familial alcoholism *per se* were controlled, then premorbid family and personality instability no longer made a statistical contribution to the risk of alcoholism."[7] He also states that "it was difficult to discard the illusion that alcohol serves as successful self-medication for unhappy, diffident people." Further, "thus core city subjects with an alcoholic parent but with an otherwise stable family were five times as likely to develop alcoholism as were subjects from clearly multiproblem families without an alcoholic parent." Numerous other studies with single drug and polydrug users have shown that when the addict is detoxified and stabilized and then is tested and examined, the incidence of major underlying psychopathology is no greater than in the population at large.

🌀 It is true many people use psychoactive drugs for a variety of reasons. The reasons why addicted and nonaddicted persons use drugs, at least in the initial stages, are the same. The difference lies in what happens when they use the drug, and this difference is qualitative. In the nonaddicted person, use of the drug diminishes the desire to use more of the drug. However, in the person with addictive disease, use of the drug fuels the desire to use more, and the desire ultimately becomes almost insatiable. Continued use, usually at high doses, will produce progressive and ultimately severe dysfunction. If the addict is psychologically tested during this phase of active use, he or she will manifest a broad spectrum of psychopathology. However, what is being evaluated at this point is a personality warped and distorted by the drug. This may lead to invalid conclusions and inappropriate treatment. I believe that individual psychotherapy is rarely appropriate for at least a year after detoxification, except in cases of severe depression or active suicidal ideation.

Finally, if the cause of addictive disease was basically psychological, then once the psyche was "back in shape," the person should be able to again use psychoactive drugs in a social way. However, experience has shown that no matter how solid the psyche, return to any "social" psychoactive drug use will rapidly lead to reinstitution of the pattern of addictive drug use with its attendant dysfunction. This tends to occur quickly, sometimes with fatal results, even after prolonged periods of sobriety.

TREATMENT CONSIDERATIONS

It is apparent from the above discussion that addictive disease is, in the words of Alcoholics Anonymous, truly "cunning, baffling and powerful," and an "equal opportunity disease," since it affects all strata of society. It is also potentially fatal, and therefore the initial thrust should be to get the person into appropriate treatment as quickly as possible. This may be inpatient or outpatient, group therapy, Alcoholics Anonymous, Narcotics Anonymous, or Cocaine Anonymous, depending on the individual's needs and the available resources.

Once the individual has entered treatment and detoxification has been completed, the more formal work of recovery should begin. I define recovery as the process of leading a comfortable and responsible life without the use of psychoactive drugs. This is a positive ongoing process which is very different than simply not using drugs. The foundation for this process is best accomplished through the Twelve Steps of A.A. or N.A.

This concept also allows us to relieve the person of some of the guilt associated with having the disease. I tell patients they are not responsible for having the disease. Nobody asked them if they wanted it. However, once they know they have the disease and what that means in terms of drug use, they are responsible for their recovery.

If one accepts the concept of addictive disease, certain other corollaries must necessarily follow. If the person is addicted to one psychoactive drug, then addiction to any other psychoactive drug is probable. This has great import for people who are willing to give up the drug which has gotten them into trouble, but who may be reluctant to give up other drugs they have not, to date, used addictively. Based on extensive clinical experience, use of any psychoactive drug will usually lead back to use of the primary drug or addiction to the secondary drug (drug switching). I believe the only safe path to follow is complete abstinence from all psychoactive drugs.

As previously noted, a family history of addictive disease increases the risk that the progeny will become addicted when exposed to the drug. Therefore, the risk is not the same for the entire population at large. This "differential risk" needs to be addressed so children of high-risk families are aware they may be at a higher risk for developing addictive disease than their peers.

Finally, this is not a position paper against psychoactive drug use. Its purpose is to clarify and delineate the concept of addictive disease so more effective treatment may become a reality.

Chapter 2
ENDNOTES

1. E .M. Jellinek, *The Disease Concept of Alcoholism,* (New Haven: College and University Press, 1960).
2. *Dorland's Illustrated Medical Dictionary,* 23rd ed. (Philadelphia: Saunders, 1957), p. 393.
3. D. W. Goodwin, *Alcoholism and Heredity, A Review and Hypothesis,* (Arch Gen Psychiatry: 1979), 36:57-61.
4. M. Buxton, and M. Jessup, unpublished study, 1982.
5. D. E. Smith, interview, Sept. 1984.
6. Mark S. Gold, *800-Cocaine,* (New York: Bantam, 1984), p. 10.
7. G. E. Vaillant, *The Natural History of Alcoholism,* (Cambridge: Harvard University Press, 1983).

3
THE MEDICAL COMPLICATIONS OF COCAINE ABUSE
Joseph C. McCarthy, M.D.

EAR, NOSE, AND THROAT

Cocaine is readily absorbed from the nasal mucosa. After intranasal administration of 1.5 mg/kg of cocaine to thirteen surgical patients, cocaine was detected in the plasma within three minutes and peak plasma concentrations were reached in 15 to 60 minutes.[1] In addition, cocaine was still detectable on the nasal mucosa up to three hours after application. The peak plasma levels attained are dose dependent with higher intranasal doses of cocaine producing higher peak plasma levels.[2] Because of its pronounced vasoconstricting properties, cocaine can cause acute and chronic rhinitis and chronic sinusitis as well as ulceration and perforation of the nasal septum.[3] Sawicka and Trosser have reported a case of cerebrospinal fluid leakage from the nose and concomitant inability to smell after cocaine sniffing, presumably due to changes in the bony portion of the skull in this area and the nerves responsible for the sense of smell.[4]

Cocaine sniffing may produce a profound rebound redness and congestion of the nasal mucosa. Chronic cocaine sniffers are also more prone to develop upper respiratory infections, and they may use a variety of nasal sprays, salt or tap water, glycerine, or Vitamin E oil to prevent or soothe irritation of the nasal mucosa. In addition, the adulterants and diluents used to cut the cocaine may also play a role in damaging the nasal mucosa. Seigel has reported dry lips and sore throats in chronic cocaine freebase smokers.[5]

Cocaine drops repeatedly instilled in the eye may cause clouding and ulcerations of the cornea, which is the reason cocaine is no longer used for eye surgery.[6] In addition, acute glaucoma may occur after topical application of cocaine to the eye. Nausea, vomiting, and vertigo have been caused by application of cocaine to the middle ear.[7] Klough has commented on the potential danger of aspiration when cocaine is applied directly to the superior laryngeal nerve or when it is applied to the nose and runs down to anesthetize the pharynx and larynx.[8]

CARDIOVASCULAR

Small doses of cocaine may slow the heart rate as a result of central vagal stimulation, but larger doses increase both heart rate and blood pressure and these effects appear to be dose related.[9] Fischman and Schuster showed that 8 mg of cocaine administered intravenously to normal, healthy volunteers increased the heart rate by 21%, and 16 mg and 32 mg increased the heart rate by 30 and 37.5% respectively. Increases in blood pressure were less striking, with an 8 mg dose of cocaine showing no change from a placebo injection and 16 mg and 32 mg showing a peak increase of approximately 15%.[10] These increases probably result from increased central sympathetic stimulation and from peripherally mediated sympathetic vasoconstriction. Conversely, a large intravenous dosage of cocaine may cause immediate death from cardiac failure due to a direct toxic action on the heart muscle.[11]

In a clinical setting, in addition to hypertension and tachycardia, cocaine has been reported to cause accelerated ventricular rhythm,[12] ventricular ectopic beats,[13] angina, a subsequent subendocardial myocardial infarction,[14] and ventricular fibrillation and death.[15] There is no consistent or definite dose at which any of the above toxic effects may occur. In Fischman and Schuster's study volunteers took up to 224 mg of cocaine intravenously over one hour with no evidence of cardiac arrhythmias or any other signs of cardiovascular toxicity. However, others have reported fatal reactions with as little as 22 mg injected submucosally.[16]

Treatment of the acute cardiovascular complications of cocaine administration should proceed in steps commensurate with the danger which the condition presents to the patient. Thus, a mild degree of hypertension and tachycardia in an otherwise healthy individual requires no pharmacological treatment. For the treatment of ventricular ectopy, lidocaine in a IV bolus of 50-100 mg, and a repeat bolus or continuous intravenous infusion at 2-4 mg/min is recommended if the ectopy continues.[17,18] If ventricular ectopy, increasing ventricular tachycardia, or hypertension persist, Propanolol may be the drug of choice.[19] This can be administered as a 1 mg IV bolus at one minute intervals up to a total of 6 mg if necessary. However, not all authorities agree that this is the drug of choice.[20] For the treatment of ventricular tachycardia in general, the *Medical Letter* recommends IV Lidocaine followed by cardioversion. If these are ineffective, bretylium (Bretlol) may be effective.[21] However, there have been no reports of the use of this regimen in ventricular tachycardia specifically due to cocaine toxicity. Obviously, other appropriate basic life supportive measures should be instituted as needed.

RESPIRATORY

Smoking cocaine, either as "pasta" (cocaine paste) or as cocaine freebase, is an extremely efficient way to quickly achieve substantial blood levels of cocaine. Jeri has reported extensively on the phenomenon of coca paste smoking in Peru.[22,23] The coca paste is a crude form of cocaine containing a number of other substances such as methanol, kerosene, sulphuric acid, etc. The paste contains 40-85% cocaine sulfate and is usually mixed with tobacco or marijuana in a cigarette. The smoking binges may last for several days and the smokers may consume as many as 50 cigarettes in one night. As a result of this prolonged and high-dose administration of cocaine, the users experience euphoria followed by dysphoria, hallucinosis, and cocaine psychosis. These states are discussed more fully in the section on central nervous system effects of cocaine.

Paly et al. have shown that plasma cocaine levels as high as 975 ng/ml can be achieved within five minutes of smoking 0.5 g of high-grade cocaine paste mixed with tobacco.[24] In a similar experiment, Paly et al.(1982) reported that plasma cocaine concentrations as high as 462 ng/ml were obtained only three minutes after subjects smoked similar combinations of high-grade cocaine paste and tobacco.[25] These levels were obtained in spite of the fact that Jeffcoat et al. have reported that an average of only 6.1% of cocaine freebase could be recovered intact from the mainstream smoke of a burning cigarette.[26] The average relative bioavailability of the cocaine is only 70% of that obtained by the nasal route. The mean half-life of cocaine by this route was 38 minutes, which is slightly shorter than has been reported for other routes of administration. The above levels and time frames are roughly equivalent to those obtained by the intravenous route.

Cocaine freebase smoking has been practiced in the United States since the early 1970s. This method of administration, probably because of decreased efficiency, allows significantly greater quantities of cocaine to be consumed than is possible through either the nasal or intravenous route. Siegel has reported that individuals may consume up to 30g per 24 hours or up to 150g in 72 hours.[27] In addition, users may smoke without interruption for extended periods of time (a *run*). In Siegel's study, the longest reported run was fourteen days. Cocaine freebase smokers always experience a progression from euphoria to dysphoria and frequently will go on to experience paranoia and psychosis. Users report a number of concurrent physical problems including dry chapped lips, sore throats, wispy voices, chest and back pains, and occasionally black and bloody sputum. It would seem reasonable to assume that they will also have an increased incidence of bronchitis, although this has not been reported.

A number of pulmonary complications from cocaine freebase use have been reported. Pneumomediastinum and pneumothorax have been reported in two young women.[28] Similar complications have been reported after marijuana smoking.[29] Miller et al. raise the possibility that the frequent, prolonged Valsalva maneuver (attempted forced expiration with the glottis closed) that illegal drug users perform may be a risk factor.[30] Weiss et al. report on two patients who smoked cocaine freebase and had a significant reduction in their pulmonary carbon monoxide diffusing capacity.[31] They hypothesize that this damage may be caused by a direct vasoconstricting effect on the pulmonary vasculature. It was not stated whether this effect was acute or did, in fact, persist. A highly unusual complication of cocaine sniffing was reported by Cooper et al., who found cellulose granulomas in the lungs.[32] In addition, Allred et al. report a fatal case of pulmonary edema in a 26-year-old man who injected cocaine freebase.[33]

GASTROINTESTINAL

Contrary to earlier reports, cocaine is well absorbed from the GI tract.[34] The peak plasma level occurs later after oral administration than after intranasal administration, perhaps because the drug is not absorbed until it reaches the alkaline milieu of the small intestine.[35] Central stimulation of the vomiting center may result in emesis just as with other methods of administration.[36] Further adrenergic stimulation may cause anorexia and/or diarrhea.

A subject of recent interest has been the cocaine *body*

packer syndrome. This refers to a method of attempting to smuggle drugs through customs. The packer, or "mule," will swallow several packets of cocaine, which are usually wrapped with latex and, once through customs, the packets are expelled and the cocaine is recovered. One of the dangers of this method of transport is massive cocaine overdose due to leakage or rupture of the packets within the intestine.[37,38] A further complication, intestinal obstruction requiring laparotomy, has also been reported.[39,40] Close medical observation and use of mild purgatives to aid in bowel evacuation appears to be the treatment of choice in the uncomplicated patient.

CENTRAL NERVOUS SYSTEM

Cocaine stimulates the central nervous system by blocking the reuptake of catecholamines from the synaptic cleft.[41] It is this reuptake process that is primarily responsible for terminating the actions of both adrenergic impulses and circulating catecholamines at adrenergic nerve endings. Therefore, since much of the neurotransmitter is left in the symaptic cleft, it will continue to stimulate the dendrites of the succeeding cell. This process will continue until the neurotransmitter is broken down enzymatically, diffuses into adjoining tissue, or is allowed to be pumped back into the cell following the breakdown of cocaine and the release of the reuptake pump. The two major neurotransmitters which appear to be active in this process are norephinephrine and dopamine, and the reinforcing and euphorigenic effects appear to be due especially to dopamine.[42] These effects can be partially blocked by Pimazole, a dopamine antagonist.

However, other mechanisms may be operative since tricyclic antidepressants also block the reuptake of catecholamines, and they do not produce euphoria nor are they common drugs of abuse. In addition, prior treatment with reserpine blocks the central effects of cocaine, but not that of amphetamines which produce psychological effects very similar to cocaine.[43]

It is possible to characterize, in a general way, the mood changes which cocaine produces in humans. However, it must be appreciated that the length and intensity of the mood states will be influenced by a number of variables including dose, method of administration, period of use, and expectations of the user.

Generally the first state to be experienced is one of pleasure which often escalates into euphoria — the cocaine high. This is often accompanied or followed by restlessness, excitement, and garrulousness. Perceptual awareness increases and the subject may become hyperaroused and hypervigilant, sometimes to the point of interpreting as hostile any rapid movement by those around him or her. A heightened grandiose sense of self as opposed to the environment is often noted.

The initial state of stimulation is followed by a rather rapid mood reversal. Anxiety and agitation become the predominant mode. The subject may become restless and irritable. Nausea and vomiting may occur. As the cocaine level continues to fall, the user may become confused, apathetic, and depressed, and experience a strong desire to use more cocaine, a behavior he or she knows will rapidly reverse the negative mood state.

The depression may be severe enough for the user to actively consider suicide. Initially, the stimulus for repeated cocaine use is the desire to recapture the cocaine high. However, as the addictive process progresses, this may be replaced by the desire to avoid the "crash," the depressing, apathetic low which occurs after cocaine use.

Chronic high dose users of cocaine may become more dysfunctional and progress to the paranoid state. Initially, this may manifest itself as free-floating suspiciousness which, with continued use, can escalate to full-blown paranoid ideation with ideas of reference. Repetitive movements, muscle twitching, and tics may be seen. If cocaine use is terminated at this point, the patient will, over time, gradually return to his or her baseline state and no additional treatment will usually be needed except treatment for the addiction itself.

The most florid psychological manifestation of cocaine toxicity is the state of cocaine psychosis. The predominant orientation is one of paranoia and may result in violent life-threatening behavior both to the subject and those around him or her. At this time, the user may experience auditory, visual, and tactile hallucinations ("snow lights" and "coke bugs"). Sleep deprivation and prolonged periods of not eating may also predispose the user to progress to the psychotic state. Some clinics have successfully treated these patients in a structured outpatient setting using haloperidol (Haldol) 2 mg orally twice a day.[44] However, for many patients, hospitalization and large doses of Haldol may be required. The psychosis itself is similar to the psychosis produced by amphetamines, but is generally shorter in duration. Users with underlying psychopathology may have more prolonged psychotic reactions. Conversely, the psychotic state may persist for months and may occur in patients with no previous personal or family history of psychosis.

As the dose of cocaine is increased, the lower centers of the brain become stimulated. Initially the rate and depth of respiration are increased. However, if the cocaine level continues to rise, the breathing may become shallow and irregular or Cheyne-Stokes respirations leading to dyspnea and cyanosis may occur. Finally, respiratory failure supervenes with central respiratory depression and unconsciousness. The hypoxia caused by the respiratory failure, in concert with cardiac arrhythmias which decrease cardiac output, may finally lead to circulatory failure and death.

Stimulation of the central nervous system may cause tonic-clonic convulsions. Obviously this effect would be potentiated by hypoxia or any compromise of the circulatory system and status epilepticus may ensue. The preferred drugs for the treatment of this condition are diazepam or a short-acting barbiturate given intravenously. The phenomenon of *kindling* (repetitive and intermittent subthreshold stimulation of the limbic system eventually leading to convulsions) has been reported in animals, but not in humans.

Increase in body temperature, sometimes to dangerous levels, may occur due to increased muscular activity and marked vasoconstriction. In addition, cocaine may act directly on the heat-regulating center in the diencephalon causing it to "reset" at a higher level. A cooling blanket or ice packs may be required to effectively combat the hyperpyrexia.

It would seem reasonable to assume that a CVA could be caused by the marked and sometimes prolonged hypertension which may occur as a result of cocaine use. This may be similar to the CVAs reported with intravenous amphetamine use. Lichtenfeld et al. have recently reported on two cases of subarachnoid hemorrhage occurring in young women minutes after they snorted cocaine. In both of these cases a congenital abnormality of the cerebral circulation was present.[45]

SEXUALITY

Cocaine use and sexual experience has rarely been studied in any scientific manner. Most of the reported experience has been anecdotal and incomplete. In the experience of Gay at the Haight-Ashbury Free Medical Clinic, cocaine would supplant all other drugs in the area of sexual enhancement because of its ability to "boost sexual eroticism."[46] Because of this property, it is highly regarded as an aphrodisiac by both the drug culture and the Peruvian Indians. Smith and Wesson report that while cocaine enhances sexual desire at low doses, higher doses, particularly in injectors or freebase users, leads to sexual dysfunction.[47] Both men and women may experience a decrease in sexual desire. In a random sample of women calling the 800-COCAINE hot line, Gold reports that 50 percent of the women reported a complete loss of sexual desire.[48] Additionally, in men there may be an impaired ability to ejaculate or maintain an erection, while in women there may be difficulty in achieving orgasm.

The sexually stimulating properties of the drug sometimes leads to adventuresome application of cocaine to the genitals. Since the drug is readily absorbed through the mucosal surface, and since it produces a profound topical anesthetic effect in the area, subsequent sexual activity may be both prolonged and intense. This, in turn, may lead to injury to the genitals. In addition, the marked stimulating properties of the drug may lead to sexual behavior such as masturbation or multipartner marathons.[49]

USE OF OTHER DRUGS WITH COCAINE

The use of depressant or "downer" drugs by cocaine users, particularly high-dose users, is common. In an attempt to counteract the dysphoric, "wired" feeling that cocaine may produce, or in order to delay, titrate, or "mellow" the crash that occurs after cocaine use, the user may add a variety of depressant drugs. This pharmacologic mixing is most common among those who use cocaine intravenously or smoke cocaine freebase. Of the depressant drugs, alcohol, narcotics, methaqualone (Quaalude), diazepam (Valium), and marijuana are most commonly used. Obviously, the use of two or more psychoactive drugs may lead to polydrug dependence or sedative dependence and complicate the withdrawal process.

The use of alcohol as a way to "come down" from cocaine is fairly common. As the dose and toxicity of cocaine use increase, progressively larger quantities of alcohol are required. Thus, it is not unusual for the high-dose cocaine user to require a fifth of hard liquor every 24 hours to keep from getting too wired while on a cocaine run. This may occur even in subjects who have not abused alcohol prior to their involvement with cocaine. The user may suffer all the consequences of high-dose alcohol abuse as well as cocaine abuse, and the combination may produce states of extreme physical and behavioral dysfunction. Therefore, in the detoxification process, pharmacotherapy for alcohol withdrawal as well as cocaine withdrawal would need to be addressed. Other downer drugs such as methaqualone and diazapam would add their own behavioral modifying properties to the cocaine and may produce additional problems of dependence and addiction.

A further problem may arise due to the addition of adulterants to the cocaine. These are drugs which have psychoactive properties of their own and are added to the cocaine in order to "cut" the drug. Drugs which have been used as adulterants include amphetamines, PCP, ephedrine, caffeine, lidocaine, and procaine. The user may be unaware that other psychoactive drugs have been added to the cocaine and thus may not be prepared to handle the effect of the resultant drug interaction.

The use of narcotics in conjunction with cocaine is a common problem with the high-dose user. Heroin, Dilaudid, Demerol, Codeine, and others have all been used to titrate the undesirable side effects of cocaine. In addition to their effects on mentation and the possibility of overdose, the combination may lead to addiction to the secondary drugs, in this case the opiate. As with the downer drugs, the medical management of the opiate withdrawal state may need to be addressed.

GENERAL COMPLICATIONS OF NONMEDICAL INTRAVENOUS DRUG USE

The intravenous cocaine user has the opportunity to experience all the complications which occur as a result of intravenous drug use. Some of the major complications are hepatitis, endocarditis, pulmonary complications such as abscess formation and pneumonia, thrombophlebitis, septic cutaneous complications, eosinophilia, hemolytic anemia, and septic arthritis. In addition, three cases of botulism have been reported.

BEHAVIORAL TOXICITY

Because of the severe mental dysfunction which often takes place, the cocaine user may be involved in home accidents such as burns incurred while preparing freebase or driving accidents while attempting to drive an automobile. In addition, the intense paranoia which occurs may lead to acts of physical violence against others. During a cocaine run, the user's all-encompassing involvement with the drug, as well as the effect of the drug itself, may lead to anorexia with poor or no food intake and lack of attention to personal hygiene. Decreased intake of food and fluid plus diarrhea may lead to dehydration and electrolyte disturbances.

UNUSUAL REACTIONS

A rare but potentially lethal condition may exist in users who have a deficiency of plasma pseuodocholinesterase, since this is the enzyme primarily responsible for the breakdown of cocaine in the body. In those users who are homozygous for the atypical serum cholinesterase, even a "normal" dose of cocaine may be fatal because they are unable to metabolize the drug appropriately.

WITHDRAWAL

Withdrawal from cocaine, by itself, tends to follow the general pattern of stimulant withdrawal much like that seen with amphetamines. Thus, the withdrawal may include lethargy, fatigue, mild muscle aches, a feeling of weakness, and some sleep disturbance. In the high-dose users, particularly those who use cocaine intravenously or smoke freebase, the above symptoms may be present to a more marked degree. In addition, there may be eating binges, subjective chills, and periods of depression. Aspirin for muscle cramps and L-tryptophan in a dose of 4 gms at bedtime for sleep have been found effective. Most withdrawal symptoms will usually disappear in three to seven days, although a low energy level and sleep disturbances may last longer. The existence of a protracted withdrawal is controversial.

It has been my experience that those patients who are not depressed and do not have a preceding history of major depression will not require the use of tricyclic antidepressant, but will simply get less depressed over time. Obviously, in cases of severe unremitting depression, antidepressant therapy and psychotherapy may be indicated. Patients who have active suicidal ideation require psychiatric hospitalization.

As during any withdrawal, active psychological support and attention to good nutrition, vitamin supplementation, and fluid balance will probably minimize the time and discomfort of the withdrawal period.

CHAPTER 3
ENDNOTES

1. C. Van Dyke, P. G. Barash, P. Jatlow, and R. Byck, "Cocaine: Plasma Concentrations after Intranasal Application in Man," *Science*, 191 (1976): 859.
2. S. H. Miller, B. Dvorchich, and T. S. Davis, *Plastic Reconstructive Surgery*, 60 (1977): 566.
3. G. R. Gay, "You've Come a Long Way, Baby! Coke Time for the New American Lady of the Eighties," *Journal of Psychoactive Drugs*, 13 (1981): 297-317.
4. E. H. Sawicha and A. Trosser, "Cerebrospinal Fluid Rhinorrhea after Cocaine Sniffing," *British Medical Journal*, 286 (1983): 1476-77.

5. R. K. Siegel, "Cocaine Freebase," *Journal of Psychoactive Drugs*, 14 (1982): 311-19.
6. K. Pearman, "Cocaine: A Review," *Journal of Laryngo Otolaryngology*, 93 (1979): 1191-99.
7. B. H. Senturia, *Journal of the American Medical Association*, 206 (1968): 1802.
8. C. A. Keogh, *Diseases of the Ear, Nose and Throat*, W. G. Brown Scott, J. Ballantyne, and J. Groves, eds. (London: Butterworth's, 1965), 170.
9. M. W. Fischman, C. R. Schuster, L. Resnekov, et al., "Cardiovascular and Subjective Effects of Intravenous Cocaine Administration in Humans," *Archives of General Psychiatry*, 33 (1976): 983-89.
10. M. W. Fischman and C. R. Schuster, "Cocaine Self-Administration in Humans," *Federation Proceedings* 41 (1982): 241-6.
11. J. M. Ritchie and N. M. Greene, "Local Anesthetics," A. S. Gilman, L. S. Goodman, and A. Gilman, eds., *The Pharmacological Basis of Therapeutics* (New York: MacMillan, 1980), 300-20.
12. A. Benchimol, H. Bartoll, and K. B. Desser, "Accelerated Ventricular Rhythm and Cocaine Abuse," *Annals of Internal Medicine*, 88 (1978): 519-20.
13. D. Young and J. J. Glauber, "Electrocardiographic Changes Resulting from Acute Cocaine Intoxication," *American Heart Journal*, 34 (1947): 272-79.
14. D. L. Coleman, T. F. Ross, and J. L. Naughton, "Myocardial Ischemia and Infarction Related to Recreational Cocaine Use," *Western Journal of Medicine*, 136 (1982):444-46.
15. C. V. Welti and R. K. Wright, "Death Caused by Recreational Cocaine Use," *Journal of the American Medical Association*, 241 (1979): 2519-22.
16. C. Van Dyke and R. Byck, "Cocaine: 1884-1974," E. H. Ellinwood and M. M. Kirby, eds., *Cocaine and Other Stimulants* (New York: Plenum, 1977), 1-30.

17. G. R. Gay, "The Deadly Delights of Cocaine," *Emergency Medicine*, (Feb. 1983): 67-81.
18. P. G. Barash, "Cocaine in Clinical Medicine," R. C. Petersen and R. C. Stillman, eds., *Cocaine: 1977* (Rockville, Md.: National Institute on Drug Abuse, 1977): DHEW publication no. (ADM) 77-471. (Research monograph series no. 13)
19. R. T. Rappolt, G. R. Gay, M. Soman, and M. Kobernich, "Treatment Plan for Acute and Chronic Adrenergic Poisoning Crises Utilizing Sympatholytic Effects of the B1-B2 Receptor Site Blocker Propranolol in Concert with Diazepam and Urine Acidification," *Clinical Toxicology*, 14 (1979): 55-69.
20. S. Cohen, *Cocaine Today* (Rockville, Md.: American Council on Marijuana and other Psychoactive Drugs, 1981).
21. "Treatment of Cardiac Arrhythmias," *The Medical Letter of Drugs and Therapy*, 25 (1983): 21-28.
22. F. R. Jeri, "The Syndrome of Coca Paste," *Journal of Psychoactive Drugs*, 10 (1978): 361-70.
23. F. R. Jeri, C. C. Sanchez, T. Del Pozo, M. Fernandez, and C. Carbajal, "Further Experience with the Syndromes Produced by Coca Paste Smoking," F. R. Jeri, ed., *Cocaine 1980. Proceedings of the International Seminar on Medical and Sociological Aspects of Coca and Cocaine* (Lima, Peru: Pacific Press, 1980), 76-85.
24. D. Paly, C. Van Dyke, P. Jatlow, F. R. Jeri, and R. Byck, "Plasma Levels after Cocaine Paste Smoking," F. R. Jeri, ed., *Cocaine 1980. Proceedings of the International Seminar on Medical and Sociological Aspects of Coca and Cocaine* (Lima, Peru: Pacific Press, 1980), 106-10.
25. D. Paly, P. Jatlow, C. Van Dyke, F. R. Jeri, R. Byck, "Plasma Cocaine Concentrations During Cocaine Paste Smoking," *Life Science*, 30 (1982): 731-38.
26. A. R. Jeffcoat, M. E. Wall, C. E. Cook, K. H. Davis, J. M. Hill, and M. B. Marr. "Stability of cocaine to pyrolytic conditions," Report to NIDA, 1980. Contract No. 271-80-3705.

27. R. K. Siegel, "Cocaine Freebase," *Journal of Psychoactive Drugs*, 13 (1982): 297-317.
28. R. Shesser, C. Davis, and S. Edelstein, "Pneumomediastinum and Pneumothorax after Inhaling Alkaloidal Cocaine," *Annals of Emergency Medicine*, 10 (1981): 213-15.
29. K. L. Mattox, "Pneumomediastinum in Heroin and Marijuana Users," *The Journal of the American College of Emergency Physicians*, 5 (1976): 36.
30. W. E. Miller, R. E. Spiekerman, and N. G. Hepper, "Pneumomediastinum Resulting from Performing the Valsalva Maneuver During Marijuana Smoking," *Chest*, 62 (1972): 233.
31. R. D. Weiss, P. D. Goldenheim, S. M. Merin, C. A. Hales, and J. H. Mendelson, "Pulmonary Dysfunction in Cocaine Smokers," *American Journal of Psychiatry*, 138 (1981): 1110-12.
32. C. B. Cooper, T. R. Bai, and E. Heyderman, "Cellulose Granulomas in the Lung of a Cocaine Sniffer," *British Medical Journal*, 286 (1983): 2021-22.
33. R. J. Allred and S. Ewer, "Fatal Pulmonary Edema Following Intravenous "'Freebase' Cocaine Use," *Annals of Emergency Medicine*, 10 (1981): 441-42.
34. C. Van Dyke, P. Jatlow, P. G. Barash, and R. Byck, "Oral Cocaine: Plasma Concentrations and Central Effects," *Science*, 200 (1978): 211.
35. K. Pearman, "Cocaine: A Review," *Journal of Laryngo Otolaryngology*, 93 (1979): 1191-99.
36. J. M. Ritchie and N. M. Greene, "Local Anesthetics," A. S. Gilman, L. S. Goodman, and A. Gilman, eds., *The Pharmacological Basis of Therapeutics* (New York: Macmillan, 1980), 300-20.
37. D. A. Fishbain and C. V. Welti, "Cocaine Intoxication, Delirium and Death in a Body Packer," *Annals of Emergency Medicine*, 10 (1981): 531-32.
38. J. Bettinger, "Cocaine Intoxication: Massive Oral Overdose," *Annals of Emergency Medicine*, 9 (1980): 429-30.

39. M. M. McCarron and J. D. Wood, "The Cocaine 'Body Packer' Syndrome." *Journal of the American Medical Association*, 250 (1983): 1417-20.
40. D. S. Caruana, B. Weinbach, D. Goerg, and L. B. Gardner, "Cocaine—Packet Ingestion," *Annals of Internal Medicine*, 100 (1984): 73-74.
41. J. M. Ritchie and N. M. Greene, "Local Anesthetics," A. S. Gilman, L.S. Goodman, and A. Gilman, eds., *The Pharmacological Basis of Therapeutics* (New York: Macmillan, 1980), 300-20.
42. J. H. Jaffe, "Drug Addiction and Drug Abuse," A. S. Gilman, L. S. Goodman, and A. Gilman, eds., *The Pharmacological Basis of Therapeutics*. (New York: Macmillan, 1980), 535-84.
43. E. H. Ellinwood, Jr., "Amphetamine Psychosis: A Multidimensional Process," *Seminars in Psychiatry*, 1 (1969): 208-26.
44. D. E. Smith, "Diagnostic, Treatment and Aftercare Approaches to Cocaine Abuse," *Journal of Substance Abuse Treatment*, 1 (1984): 5-9.
45. P. J. Lichtenfeld, D. B. Rubin, and R. S. Feldman, "Subarachnoid Hemorrhage Precipitated by Cocaine Snorting," *Archives of Neurology*, 41 (1984): 223-24.
46. Gay, "You've Come a Long Way, Baby!" 297-317.
47. Smith, "Diagnostic, Treatment and Aftercare Approaches to Cocaine Abuse," 5-9.
48. "Women's Cocaine Use Rising." *The U.S. Journal of Drug and Alcohol Dependence,* (May 1984).
49. Smith, "Diagnostic, Treatment and Aftercare Approaches to Cocaine Abuse," 5-9.

4
THE STYLES OF ENABLING BEHAVIOR
Charles E. Nelson, Ph.D.

INTRODUCTION

Gottleib's book, *The Pleasures of Cocaine*,[1] opens with the following "Introductory Statements on the Author's Attitude Toward Cocaine Use:"

> It is the personal political philosophy of the author that the adult individual has a biological birthright which allows him [or her] the freedom to be sovereign of his own mind and body and that he may do with himself anything that he pleases. . . . Properly interpreted and applied, the right of personal sovereignty should include the right to take into one's own body any substance one desires, whether it be for nutritional, medicinal, psychedelic or hedonistic purposes.

Aside from a brief suggestion about not directly infringing upon the rights of others, no comment was made about the sovereignty and the freedom of those who are intimately entangled in this person's life. Few cocaine abusers live in a void. The rights of spouses, children, lovers, friends, or even parents are directly and indirectly infringed upon.

Cocaine abusers routinely engender confusion, dysphoria, and distress in those who are the most intimately entangled in their lives. In response, these significant others often develop pathological coping strategies and defense mechanisms parallel to the cocaine abusers and thus have been given the behavioral descriptor *codependents*. Many of the spouses or lovers of cocaine abusers use the drug themselves, and are behaviorally described as *user codependents* or *coaddicts*. Although codependents do not cause abuse of the cocaine, they often support the progressive development of the abusive behavior. The drug treatment community has labeled this support of the chemical abuse *enabling*. The label *enabler* has not received broad acceptance from the treatment community, but the behavioral descriptor enabling has gained wide use and acceptance.

ROOTS OF PATHOLOGY WITHIN THE RELATIONSHIP SYSTEM

The influence of the cocaine abuser upon the codependents is not a one-way street. The pathological influences become a major part of the dynamics of the entire cocaine abuser/codependent system of relationships. Murray Bowen's family systems theory illustrated the dynamics of these influences. He used the human body to analogize how a change in the functioning of one member is automatically followed by a compensatory change in another member of the system. He pointed out that the body has an intricate set of balancing mechanisms to deal with changes in such vital functions as temperature, reflexes, heart rate, respiration, and digestion. He suggested that

> systems function at all levels of efficiency, from robust health to total failure. There are healthy compensated functioning states in which an organ can increase its functioning to handle an increased work load. There are situations in which one organ increases its function to compensate for the poor functioning of another organ. There are states of dysfunction that range from the short-term illness to permanent dysfunction in an organ system. An organ that functions for another for long periods of time does not return to normal so easily.[2]

Bowen continued:

> There are situations of decompensated overfunctioning in which a failing organ works faster and faster in a futile effort to overcome a work overload. An example is the racing of a worn-out heart as it approaches total failure. The same patterns of function, overfunction and dysfunction are present in the way people relate to each other in families and small social systems.

How does cocaine abuse fit into Bowen's family systems concept? Although no literature was found tying cocaine abuse to this model, it was easily applied. As a dysfunction, cocaine abuse is an imbalance in functioning within the total cocaine abuser/codependents relationship system. Every member of the cocaine abuse system plays a part in the dysfunction of the dysfunctional member.

Borrowing from Virginia Satir, Wegscheider suggested that to understand the balancing phenomenon of the system, an analogy of the principles of a mobile can be applied:

> A mobile is an art form made up of rods and strings upon which are hung various parts. The beauty of the mobile is in its balance and flexibility. The mobile has a way of responding to changing circumstances such as wind. It changes position but always maintains connections with each part. If I flick one of the suspended parts and give it kinetic energy, the whole system moves to gradually bring itself to equilibrium.[3]

The same is true of the cocaine abuser/codependents system. Where there is stress, the whole system shifts to maintain equilibrium or stability. Each codependent is affected by the increasing dysfunction of the cocaine abuser and each deals with the growing pathology of the cocaine abuser by developing behavioral characteristics that cause the least immediate personal stress. These behavioral characteristics help cope with the pain of being emotionally rejected in favor of the drug.

At this point the codependents begin to clearly exhibit a personality transfiguration commonly seen in the cocaine abuser. Long-standing personal standards of behavior and value systems deteriorate and are contradicted by the codependents. They experience fears parallel to those of the cocaine abuser: anxiety, self-hatred, helplessness, hurt, loneliness, low self-worth, and guilt.[4]

Family members attempt to find some way to deal with the pain, but rarely find healthy ways to cope with the drug abuse. Eventually, they are rewarded because survival behavior, although dysfunctional and pathological, becomes a source of recognition for the codependents. Their pain is eventually blocked by several defense mechanisms, especially denial, repression, rationalization, and projection, and they become further entangled in their self-deception. These are the precursors for the enabling behavior. Without such enabling, cocaine abusers would usually suffer the consequences of their behavior.

Recently, empirical research has discovered six separate styles of enabling behavior which are commonly displayed by codependents: (1) Avoiding and Shielding, (2) Attempting to Control, (3) Taking over Responsibilities, (4) Rationalizing, (5) Cooperating and Collaborating, and (6) Rescuing and Subserving.[5] An extensive review of the literature revealed that the discovery of these styles of enabling was a pertinent and natural step following the contributions of others, maintaining continuity with the observational and theoretical groundwork on enabling behaviors laid out by the early pioneers in this field such as Virginia Satir and Murray Bowen.

The definition for the term *enabling* includes a superstructure of perspectives which many people relate to in terms of their own personal treatment orientations. The word was not created for the chemical dependency treatment field; it was transplanted. The most important factors of its transplantation were the techniques many early theorists utilized in defining their perspectives of the word. It appeared most of these theorists identified examples of enabling behavior and consequently helped elucidate parameters for the word in the context of the codependent/chemical abuser relationship.

Yet, no single definition for enabling is agreed upon, or likely ever shall be. The recent study on the styles of enabling took the next important step and established a new empirical tool, the "Cocaine Abuse Enabling Questionnaire"[6] for assessing the many ways in which enabling can be expressed. In creating this instrument, further practical examples of enabling were identified. As additional practical tools for understanding the destructive enabling styles become empirically developed, the comprehensive treatment milieu will have refined, accessible methods for assessing and treating nonuser and user codependents of cocaine abusers.

ROOTS AND DYNAMICS OF THE STYLES OF ENABLING

Enabling behaviors flourish under the cloak of several disguises or styles within the codependent/cocaine abuser system. The six styles of enabling derived from the literature are defined below.

1. *Avoiding and Shielding.* Any behavior by the codependent covering up for, or preventing the abuser, or self from experiencing the full impact of harmful consequences of drug use.

2. *Attempting to Control.* Any behavior by the codependent performed with the intent to take personal control over the significant other's drug use.

3. *Taking over Responsibilities.* Any behavior by the codependent designed to take over the abuser's personal responsibilities, such as household chores or employment.

4. *Rationalizing and Accepting.* Any behavior by the codependent conveying a rationalization or acceptance of the significant other's drug use.

5. *Cooperating and Collaborating.* Any assistance or involvement by the codependent in the buying, selling, adulterating, testing, preparing, or use of drugs.

6. *Rescuing and Subserving.* Any behavior by the codependent overprotecting the abuser and subjugating himself or herself.

The following statements made by codependents are drawn from a correlational/cluster analysis. Statistical analysis suggests that these are examples of the six enabling styles.

Avoiding and Shielding

1. I made up excuses to avoid social contact during abusive time periods.
2. I threw away, hid, or destroyed my partner's cocaine stash or paraphernalia.
3. I threatened physical violence to get my partner to quit.
4. I shielded my partner from a crisis which could have forced him or her into therapy.
5. I helped my partner keep appearances up or covered-up around relatives, friends, neighbors, or his or her employer.

Attempting to Control

1. I bought things for my partner which might divert him or her from cocaine use (sports gear, tools, car, home, etc.).
2. I spent the night at a hotel or motel to try to get my partner to quit.
3. I spent the night at a friend's or relative's house to try to get my partner to quit.
4. I stayed home from work to take care of my partner's problems resulting from cocaine.

5. I began constantly reminding or preaching to my partner about his or her failure in order to alarm him or her about the personal effects of the cocaine abuse.
6. I screamed, yelled, swore, or cried in an attempt to get my partner to stop the abuse.
7. I threatened to hurt myself in an attempt to get my partner's attention to quit.
8. I stayed away from home as much as possible to get away from it all.
9. I told my partner to leave me until he or she quit the abuse, but then immediately went looking for him or her.
10. I used or withheld sex as a way to control my partner's abuse of cocaine.

Taking over Responsibilities

1. I always woke my partner in time for work.
2. I began to do my partner's chores.
3. I began paying all the bills.
4. I covered my partner's bad checks.

Rationalizing and Accepting

1. I believed and/or communicated that the use of cocaine was safer than other drugs.
2. I rationalized and/or communicated that my partner's use of cocaine helped us to maintain ties to a group of people of a high-income level.
3. I believed and/or communicated that my partner's use of cocaine helped him or her to be more confident.
4. I believed and/or communicated that my partner's use of cocaine helped him or her to be more open.
5. I provided nose drops, nasal spray, Vitamin E, warm water, or other "aids" to soothe my partner's sore or stuffed nasal linings.
6. I believed and/or communicated that my partner's use of cocaine helped him or her to communicate better.

7. I believed and/or communicated that my partner's use of cocaine helped him or her to be happier or less depressed.
8. I believed and/or communicated that my partner's use of cocaine helped him or her to be more sexually experimental.
9. I rationalized and/or communicated that the cocaine gave my partner more alertness, creativity, clearer thinking, studying powers, or any other function aiding his or her mental activities.
10. I rationalized and/or communicated that the cocaine gave my partner more energy, endurance, coordination, or any other function aiding his or her performance in physical activities.

Cooperating and Collaborating

1. I helped my partner take the cocaine (blowing it up his or her nose or mouth, injecting him or her, lighting the pipe, etc.).
2. I helped my partner to adulterate (cut), counterfeit rocks or flakes, or reconstitute cocaine.
3. I helped my partner to adulterate (cut), counterfeit rocks or flakes, or reconstitute cocaine in my home.
4. I helped my partner weigh or package cocaine.
5. I helped my partner keep accounting records of cocaine sales.
6. I helped my partner to chop, crush, or screen his or her cocaine.
7. I helped my partner to wash, clean, or purify his or her cocaine.
8. I made available to my partner any paraphernalia for taking or preparing cocaine.
9. I supplied my partner with alcohol, tranquilizers, narcotics, or any "downers" to counterbalance the tension or agitation from cocaine.
10. I loaned or gave money to my partner for cocaine.

Rescuing and Subserving

1. I cleaned up my partner's cocaine paraphernalia when they were left out.
2. I found myself checking or measuring my partner's cocaine stash to determine how much he or she had been using.
3. I cleaned up my partner's vomit after an abusive episode.
4. I encouraged my partner to use the drug at home so he or she wouldn't get into more problems away from home.
5. I began waiting hand and foot on my partner.

The cocaine abuser's behavior may or may not be destructive in the early stages of drug use. Eventually, the consequences of the increasingly irresponsible or unhealthy behavior may become overwhelming. Awareness of this is often dulled though, since he or she rarely comes face-to-face with these consequences.

The codependents shield the cocaine abuser from those consequences and help to avoid the crises with elaborate protection systems. The blow of the crises is deflected by such *avoiding and shielding* behaviors, and problems are minimized and diverted for the moment. The cycle continues and the crises that could cause the cocaine abuser to enter a chemical dependency treatment program are obstructed. Any isolated act of enabling is less important than the harmful patterns which emerge.

If the behavior is so destructive, why do codependents choose to continue the enabling? They perceive all of their behavior as sincere efforts in helping. Whatever style or combination of styles a codependent applies, the decisions are made under duress, without any knowledge of the effects. The enabling of cocaine abuse is naively done either with genuine concern or self-preservation in mind.

At first, codependents may not perceive the abusive episodes or chronic cocaine abuse as destructive; yet, they still try to comprehend why the individual acts in such confusing ways. Rather than understanding the behavior as an outgrowth of chemical dependency, they may *rationalize and accept* it as coping behavior. At this point, the codependents may come to believe the abuser's confusing behavior with cocaine will go away as soon as the other stresses (work problems, depression, financial strain, family tension, and so on) disappear. They become more exposed to the potential of developing the same delusions and defense mechanisms as the cocaine abuser. The codependents' behaviors begin to support a mutual misconception of the real nature of the problem.

More serious stages ensue. The codependents' constant rationalizing and accepting of the cocaine abuser's behavior may be discredited by outsiders as "wishful thinking" or "gullibility," but eventually, chemical dependency treatment staff have the opportunity to recognize the classic symptoms of repression, rationalization, and denial. The enabling styles are in full view when the codependents begin *taking over responsibilities* of the cocaine abuser. The abuser is now left with fewer such responsibilities and his or her abusive behavior becomes further protected.

If a codependent's primary style is *attempting to control,* then anyone unfamiliar with the symptoms of enabling may view the person as doing everything he or she can to discourage the problem. Yet, all such behavior usually makes it possible for the cocaine abuse to continue. The abuser will use these behaviors as excuses to continue to use more.

CODEPENDENTS' PERSONAL ACCOUNTS

Most of the cocaine abusers and their codependents I've treated over the past ten years have discussed the personal pain and anguish caused by the behaviors surrounding cocaine abuse. Many of the codependents who also used cocaine reported the mutual use of the drug initially attracted the couple to each other, and most described how the continued use eventually destroyed the relationship. One user codependent's account of this follows:

Cocaine brought us together and it took us apart. I was probably part of the reason he got hooked and I felt guilty. Cocaine made us feel good at first and gave us something to do together. But, then. . .if I hadn't demanded that we do other recreational things, coke would be all we'd do.

Another user codependent said:

We both knew cocaine sucked, but continued nonetheless, of course. Wow, she is still doing it after quitting. She left me when I got clean and she couldn't. She became a classic coke whore.

A third user codependent told of her own reluctant involvement and eventual rejection of the drug:

My partner was totally aware of my extreme dislike of what cocaine had done to me since he introduced the drug to me. He continued to push it on me after I had quit several times. I finally gave in, mainly since I knew he would do it anyway, even if I refused. I finally drew the line and said I quit. It was then that he started not coming home after work until three a.m., two or three times a week. My reaction was hurt and rage at being left alone, not knowing if he was possibly hurt or just drinking and snorting again.

One user codependent painfully described her own confusion and entanglement with the drug and her partner:

I felt that he used it as a substitute for me. I used to confront him with, "Which is more important, me or the drug?" Often, he had no answer. When I was with him, I didn't do much coke because it repulsed me (when I saw what it did to him), but two months after we broke up I began abusing cocaine myself for about six months. So many people, when using coke, become controlled by it, get extremely selfish, and will do anything to get more.

> Cocaine, without a doubt, was the primary reason our relationship dissolved. I still think I'm scared of my own tendency to abuse it. If I had money, I'd spend it on coke. Even after all I've been through, I confess that I'd still like to shoot it, and someday will. I've got to know what that feeling was that took complete control of him and that feeling that replaced me.

The influence of enabling behavior was evident throughout many of the codependent's remarks. One nonuser codependent discussed how she began dealing cocaine, believing that it would save the family money. She felt that her dealing *(cooperating and collaborating)* prevented the rest of the family members from suffering the financial strain of her husband's buying single grams from a dealer. She went on to say:

> This way I and our daughter wouldn't be out on a limb. I quit dealing when I was about six months pregnant with our next child. I laid down the rule that it wasn't done in the house, and I didn't want to see any of it. . .so I didn't see him either.

At times only one style of enabling behavior was evident, and at other times several styles combined went on unabated. A codependent discussed the ensuing confusion:

> My partner was abusing cocaine, but I never turned him away from the drug because I didn't want him to sneak around behind my back. At least this way he stayed home and I knew exactly where he was, although he wasn't much company. He spent most of the time looking out windows and not saying anything. Also, I had to make excuses for him to bill collectors. I hated having to lie, but it was a choice between my husband or telling relatives what he was into and where our money went. I would never have to work if there was no coke, but since he ran up debts, I had to get a job.

One user codependent simply said she would use coke just so her partner couldn't do as much and it really made her unhappy about herself. Other user codependents wrote about how their use of cocaine or other drugs compromised their values and opened the door to their cooperating and collaborating style of enabling. As one of these individuals stated:

> At the times of the worst abuse — although I knew cocaine was destroying our marriage and my husband's good sense and physical health — I still condoned and helped the drug abuse because I had my own habit to deal with. As long as he had coke, he didn't bug me about my abuse and we got along fine. But it hurt me to my heart to see a good man and decent human being torn apart by cocaine. At this time we're not together . . . he's burned out now. I partially blame my abuse for allowing him to destroy himself. I could have helped.

Another codependent suffered other personal consequences as a result of her enabling:

> I told him I didn't really care about his cocaine abuse as long as he didn't bring it into the home (because of the children). He'd been in and out of jail many times, because he'd get busted at friends' houses, so I finally told him he might as well do it at home . . . that way he'd be at home and not in jail. Now we're both in jail.

One young woman's entanglement with her cocaine-abusing partner illustrates the parallel pathology of many user codependents:

> My partner went into great debt because of his cocaine use, but because I am a student I didn't have the funds to help him with his financial problems. Whenever we argued about his coke use, his view was, Why should I stop doing something that is so incredibly sexual and feels so good? He told me in vivid detail about the instant

eroticism that happens when injecting coke. I tried to insist that he shoot me up so he could look at himself differently. He wouldn't do it. He did want to share the experience with me and have me carry out erotic acts, and I tried to be a part of it, but I couldn't. He turned into a different person — eyes glaring, blood dripping from his arm. It was scary and disgusting. The use of cocaine put a huge dent in our sexual life, yet it's hard to stay away from something that makes you feel that good.

The following behavior is common among many codependents and reflects the ingenious, yet artless facade in which enabling can be concealed: "Sometimes the only way to get hubby off his ass to mow the lawn, run an errand, or anything else besides vegetate in front of the television is to get him a line."

Several of the codependents have said, as they entered treatment, they simply did not have enough information and did not know what to do. As one nonuser codependent stated:

I know very little about drugs, and I suffered because I truly cared for a person who I believe is an addict. He's been hiding his addiction until now because he thinks it's fashionable to do it. Lately, he has left me for months at a time and has gravitated to women who "party" with him. I don't know what to do.

Another nonuser codependent discussed this common feeling of helplessness which seemed to plague all of the codependents who lacked knowledge of a direction in which to turn:

I feel you should know that because of my ignorance about drugs, I was unaware of what was going on and what to do. I don't understand behavior changes and what to look for, other than a runny nose and a loss of appetite. He never had an appetite loss and I thought the nasal problems were allergy related. We are now in the process of a divorce as a result of the damage done and the psychological hell I had to relate to and deal with. I can't live with the swings in behavior. It's pure hell because I really love this man, but his behavior has become torture to me. I need to be educated about cocaine and my role.

Most of these individuals echoed this sense of confusion and a lack of knowledge about how to deal with a cocaine-abusing partner.

RECOVERING CODEPENDENTS AND TREATMENT IMPLICATIONS

Drug abuse has been commonly referred to as a progressive family disease. Byrne and Holes described this disease as a

> progressively dysfunctional lifestyle. . .not a disease which exists within people — rather, it is a disease which people exist (live) within. . .which means they can recover. The primary key to recovery is the discovery of the way to move them out of the diseased lifestyle into a new and functional lifestyle.[7]

For years it was felt that the only effective way to help cocaine abusers was to wait until they sought help on their own after "hitting bottom." Yet, the denial, repression, and rationalizations still carried many cocaine abusers right into self-destruction, losing family, possessions, friends, jobs, self-esteem, health, or life.

Treatment programs have found hitting bottom could also mean the cocaine abuser has experienced a crisis frightening or painful enough that he or she will do just about anything to avoid it — even stop snorting, injecting, or orally administering cocaine. Twenty-five years ago, Johnson[8] suggested such a crisis could be created by the codependents and it could be done before the abuser destroyed his or her life. The process of creating such a crisis was termed an *intervention*. The specific steps in the intervention process are clearly spelled out in the literature and will not be reported here. Yet, it is important to note the effectiveness of this approach is variable depending upon the skill level of the intervention specialists, the readiness of the back-up treatment program for the cocaine abuser, and availability of an equally efficacious treatment program for the codependents.

It has become clear that no treatment program could be called complete or comprehensive unless it had a component dealing with the specific issues of the codependents. "We are now at a point in the evolution of treatment. . .where it is necessary to establish acceptable standards for care not only of the identified patient but also of the significant other person."[9]

Some chemical dependency treatment programs still retain an attitude of resistance about including codependents in treatment. Program staff back away from codependent treatment for various reasons: their patients did not have codependents, codependents would not participate in treatment, or involving codependents could "upset the recovering abuser." It has been suggested that these excuses of unavailability and lack of cooperation of the codependents are simply resistances of the staff, who are reluctant about or fear doing family therapy.[10] It is possible these treatment program staff members were engaging in their own enabling behaviors.

If the cocaine abuser enters a chemical dependency treatment program where there is no active codependent education and treatment component and aftercare support system, the recovery process can be sabotaged by further enabling behaviors after the patient is discharged. Without concurrent treatment, the codependents may not accept (consciously or unconsciously) the recovering cocaine abuser as a dependable or credible financial manager, decision maker, or person capable of giving emotional support.

Even if codependents are included in the intervention and treatment stages, they may continue destructive enabling behavior. They may choose not to participate at all. Jean Caldwell is the adult counseling supervisor for the McDonald Center at Scripp's Memorial Hospital. Caldwell pointed out:

> A common comment by many codependents during treatment is, "What if he or she doesn't love me straight?" Many codependents began to perceive that their only consistent source of self-esteem came through the enabling behavior. They became reluctant to give up the "survival" behavior.[11]

Codependents may see their involvement as a defeat and an indictment of their "failures." Having lost a lucid view of their own identity, they begin to focus on the cocaine abuser rather than themselves. After living with the cocaine abuser's symptoms, which might have included lying, criminal behavior, and other forms of acting-out, the codependent may truly believe that the recovering abuser is actually not recovering and is instead purposely hiding these behaviors. Codependents may try to pressure the treatment staff to accept this perspective. Codependents may feel that the cocaine abuser should be "punished" somehow in the treatment program rather than "rewarded" by way of peer group activities, recreation, and self-esteem building exercises. The codependents may engage in anxiety-producing behavior by focusing on what will happen if the treatment "does not work." Threats of divorce if the patient isn't "fixed" by the time of discharge may occur. The codependent may panic and assign "treatment failure clues" to minute behaviors of the recovering cocaine abuser, such as appearances of a bad mood, displays of differences of opinion, or negative comments.[12] Thus, after long periods of hopelessness due to repeated failures, codependents often have a difficult time during the recovery process in not anticipating a recurrence of the past behavior.

Even if some or all of the codependents do participate in treatment and their own recovery,

> they are probably a long way from accepting him (the recovering chemical abuser) back into their midst with open arms. Even if they wanted to do this, they could not, because there are just too many past resistances in the way. There are a great many hostile feelings relating to the chemical experience, sometimes on the surface and sometimes hidden very deep.[13]

Several of these hostile feelings are aimed specifically at the role changes and expectations the recovery program has for both the recovering codependents and cocaine abusers. These role changes have a direct effect on the new lifestyle these people will build for themselves as their recovery program progresses. This period of role rebalancing commonly occurs during a time when all members of the recovering system are still burdened with residues of remorse and guilt. Other problems may still be there: financial conflicts, angry cocaine dealers, depression, acting-out children, spouses fighting. The only real change may be that the person is not actively abusing cocaine any longer.

One treatment manual pointed out that the members of the recovering abuser/codependent system "do not know what constructive communication looks or sounds like" at this time since they do not have a model. It is as though the no-talk rule has been lifted, yet no one knows the tools necessary to get the communication started. So they continue in their "noncommunication" roles in dealing with their post-treatment problems. The treatment manual closed with the suggestion:

> The pattern must change in order for the (system) to continue to recover in all areas — not just to keep the patient from using chemicals, but to learn to communicate and get back in touch with their own feelings (and deal

with their sadness, as well as their anger and frustration). There must be recovery for all members. This can be accomplished best by seeking help from outside . . . posttreatment family counseling.[14]

With the education and insight gained from intervention, treatment, and aftercare, the recovering codependents can start to deal with the recovering cocaine abuser constructively. They can stop *shielding* the other person from the consequences of his or her behavior. Through new communication tools, they can directly verbalize their concerns and discontinue their habituated styles of enabling.

Hence, when nonuser and user codependents enter the treatment process, whether alone or with the cocaine abuser, they generally are in a confused state consisting of a blend of anger, guilt, frustration, exhaustion, embarrassment, loneliness, fear, distrust, irritation, grief, and relief. It is important for treatment teams to be prepared to handle codependents as people who are experiencing the simultaneous existence of mutually conflicting feelings and thoughts about treatment. This ambivalence will be both similar to, and divergent from, the cocaine abusers' reactions to entering treatment. Both nonuser and user codependents have likely spent a great deal of time, money, and energy in their attempts to help the cocaine abuser. Even the user codependents' efforts backfired and left them with lowered self-esteem. The destructive behaviors surrounding the abuse of cocaine exert a very potent shaping influence on the personality of the codependents. Both nonuser and user codependents develop such close contact with the pathological coping mechanisms that they lose touch with their own identity. Thus, self-disclosure to the treatment team becomes difficult for most of them.

Consequently, the treatment staff may be unsure as to what style of enabling the codependent has been utilizing. One tool for discovering which style is predominant is to note how the codependent relates to the treatment team. Is the codependent *attempting to control* the staff by using threats such as, "If you don't clean him up, I'm divorcing him"? Is the codependent *taking over responsibilities* of the staff? Is the codependent *avoiding* the treatment team? Is the codependent *rescuing* the staff members? These and many other clues can aid in assessing codependents' familiar style of enabling.

Unfortunately, untrained treatment staff members have wielded the term *enabling* in a harmful way. For a few, the term has become judgmental finger-pointing, rather than an educational tool pointing the finger in constructive directions for codependents and cocaine abusers to find further answers to deal with their dilemma. When codependents exhibit the enabling styles to an untrained staff member, they often receive reactions which appear condescending or rejecting. Such attitudes can become blockades between the codependents and the treatment staff member, and need to be dealt with at the individual supervision and program in-service training levels.

When codependents do not feel blamed and are welcomed and encouraged to join in the recovery process, they usually participate. When they see a program they can identify with and educational programs which meet their needs, they stay involved. This is where treatment of codependents begins.

Chemical dependency treatment programs need to incorporate education about the styles of enabling into their in-service training. As a result, treatment teams will have potent tools to synchronously educate recovering codependents about potentially destructive behavior and allow the therapy to achieve its maximum effect. Treatment programs can upgrade their educational components to help recovering codependents recognize such behaviors and understand how they can detach from enabling, therefore positively influencing the cocaine abusers' steps in getting "clean."

Such education can allow recovering codependents to separate the destructive aspects of their enabling styles from their genuine motivation to aid the cocaine abuser. When codependents do not have tools for assessing their enabling styles, and when they do not have methods for dealing with the stresses inherent in relinguishing such acquired conduct, they may become discouraged and obstruct the therapy process. With the new knowledge gained from the education recommended above, the recovering codependents of cocaine abusers can move on within the treatment program and gain the other available benefits necessary for leading more meaningful lives.

Treatment programs should help recovering codependents understand that they may earnestly do everything suggested in the program and that the cocaine abuse still might go unchecked. However, codependents can be taught that if they are willing to learn about the styles of enabling and work on their own program of recovery, the chances of the cocaine abuser recovering are greatly increased.

Just as codependents are not responsible for their partners' abuse of cocaine, they are also not responsible for the abuser's abstinence from cocaine. Joseph Kellermann analogized recovery to the construction of a Gothic arch: "There are unseen foundations, many persons may lay various stones in the arch,"[15] but the recovery structure comes crumbling down if the keystone for the arch is not put into place by the cocaine abuser. This cannot be done by the recovering codependent. For genuine success, decisions must be made and action taken by the recovering cocaine abusers themselves.

It is the personal philosophy of this author that adults have a responsibility to balance their own rights (mind and body) with the rights of others, such as their spouse, children, lovers, or friends. Properly interpreted and applied, the right of personal sovereignty should also take into account the familial and social context in which the cocaine abuse occurs.

Chapter 4
ENDNOTES

1. Adam Gottleib, *The Pleasures of Cocaine,* (Manhattan Beach, CA: Twentieth Century Alchemist, 1981) pp. 17-19.
2. Murray Bowen, "Alcoholism as Viewed through Family Systems Theory and Family Psychotherapy." Paper presented at the Annual Meeting, National council of Alcoholism, Washington, D.C., April 3, 1973.
3. Sharon Wegscheider, *The Family Trap. . .No One Escapes From a Chemically Dependent Family,* (Minneapolis: The Johnson Institute, 1976) p. 2.
4. L. Schulamith, et al., "Effects of Alcoholism on the Family System," *Health and Social Work,* 4 (November 1979) pp. 111-27.
5. Charles Nelson, *Styles of Enabling in the Codependents of Cocaine Abusers,* (San Diego: United States International University, 1984).
6. Charles Nelson, *The Cocaine Abuse Enabling Questionnaire* (San Diego: United States International University, 1984).
7. M. M. Byrne and J. H. Holes, "The 'Co-Alcoholic' Syndrome." *Labor-Management Alcoholism Journal* 9, no. 2 (1979): pp. 68-74.
8. V. E. Johnson, *I'll Quit Tomorrow,* (New York: Random House, 1960). Available through Hazelden Educational Materials. Order no. 8021.
9. J. P. Conway, "Significant Others Need Help, Too. Alcoholism Treatment Is Just As Important to the Rest of the Family," *Focus on Alcohol and Drug Issues* 4, no.3 (May/June 1981) pp. 17-19.
10. Ibid.
11. J. Caldwell, Personal communication, La Jolla, CA, January 19, 1983.
12. Conway, 1981.

13. Johnson Institute Staff, *Recovery of Chemically Dependent People,* (Minneapolis: Johnson Institute, n.d.) p. 6.
14. Ibid, p. 8.
15. J. L. Kellermann, *A Guide for the Family of the Alcoholic,* (New York: Al-Anon Family Group Headquarters, n.d.). Available through Hazelden Educational Materials. Order no. 1300.

5
COCAINE RECOVERY SUPPORT GROUPS: THE LANGUAGE OF RECOVERY

Paul Ehrlich, M.A.
Maureen McGeehan, M.S.W., A.C.S.W.

INTRODUCTION

The purpose of this chapter is to illustrate that cocaine abuse is treatable with techniques similar to — if not identical to — approaches utilized in the treatment of other chemical dependency problems. It will describe the cocaine recovery support groups we have developed over the past four years. Within these groups, we have blended the Twelve Step concept of Alcoholics Anonymous with reality-oriented therapeutic techniques. We believe the cocaine recovery support group provides a useful model of treatment and recovery for people with cocaine dependency problems.

We began the first cocaine recovery support group in March, 1981, in response to a dramatic increase in cocaine abuse. A second group was begun in March, 1982, and two more were added during the next year to meet increased client demand. Since August 1982, we have also cofacilitated a group with the Haight-Ashbury Training and Education Project, a section of the Haight-Ashbury Free Medical Clinic (H.A.F.M.C.). In four years we have seen a total of 136 clients in these cocaine-specific groups.

DESCRIPTION OF THE GROUPS

Each cocaine recovery support group has eight to twelve members, ranging in age from nineteen to 58 years. Most members are in their late 20s and early 30s. About 60% of each group is male. The minimum level of education is high school, and several members are currently students or hold graduate and professional degrees. All members are employed at least part-time; occupations include law, music, medicine, business, homemaking, and skilled trades.

Generally, group members sought treatment following some crisis in their lives which they recognized as being caused by their cocaine use (e.g., financial problems, arrest, pressure from family or significant others). A life-threatening or frightening experience following cocaine use is a frequent precipitant, as is the repeated experience of loss of control. Most clients had made unsuccessful attempts to limit or stop cocaine use on their own.

Clients learn about our groups in a variety of ways: other clients, family members who have researched treatment options, referral from community resources, and public education presentations in the media.

Sixty-two percent of the group members are intranasal cocaine users, 26% are freebase smokers, and 12% inject the drug. Patterns of abuse vary from daily maintenance use to periodic binges of several days or weeks duration. Dosage ranges from 1-1/2 grams per week to 4 grams per day, with some members reporting much higher dosages during binge periods (up to 17 grams in a 24 hour period for high-dose freebase smokers). Though most group members report some use of other drugs, (e.g., alcohol, marijuana, Valium, methaqualone, or heroin), they usually identify cocaine use as the major source of their financial, emotional, and interpersonal problems. As treatment progresses it becomes apparent that some clients are addicted to one or more of these substances in addition to cocaine. Use of drugs other than cocaine will be subsequently discussed.

All groups are cofacilitated by a male and female counselor. The ground rules for group membership include the following:
1. agreement that identities of members and content of group discussions are held in strict confidence by all members, i.e., not discussed with anyone outside the group;
2. agreement that no one will attend a group session while under the influence of any psychoactive substance (no use in the preceding 24 hours). Occasional exceptions have been made for certain prescription medications when a proper medical diagnosis has been made;
3. an expressed desire for recovery, which is defined as "the ability to live comfortably and responsibly without the use of any psychoactive substance."

Although abstinence is not required for clients to join the group, it is the initial treatment goal. Those who do not achieve abstinence or exhibit a sincere desire for recovery are consistently challenged by their peers and tend to drop out of treatment within the first two or three months. In two instances counselors have terminated treatment for clients who failed to work toward this goal.

Some groups have developed additional agreements such as punctual attendance or more active participation in the group process.

TREATMENT PHILOSOPHY

Direct clinical experience validates recent findings that cocaine is a powerful and tenaciously addictive drug.[1] Our philosophy of treatment is based on a model of addictive disease whose symptoms are compulsion, loss of control, and continued use despite adverse consequences. Most of the psychological and social disturbances which accompany the addiction are secondary to the drug itself and not a symptom of underlying psychopathology. Symptoms related to the addiction are progressive, predictable, and potentially fatal if not treated. If drug use continues, physical health deteriorates and the ability to function in employment and interpersonal relationships gradually erodes. Self-esteem is damaged as a result. The accumulation of drug effects causes further affective and cognitive distortion. In the most severe cases toxic psychosis or death will ensue.

Recovery from addictive disease is a reversal of these processes. Recovery is in progress when the chemically dependent person has the capacity to abstain from cocaine and other drugs, to demonstrate personal freedom and responsibility, to realize personal growth and change, and to maintain meaningful and effective relationships with others.

Three basic tenets underlie all of the specific techniques or therapeutic practices employed in the groups:
1. addiction is a disease which has its basis in genetic factors, learned experience, and environmental conditioning;
2. recovery is possible;
3. while people may not be responsible for their addiction (due to a genetic predisposition or extreme compulsion produced by the drug itself), they *are* responsible for their recovery.

The cocaine recovery support groups encourage clients to achieve the following long-term goals:
1. abstinence from mood-altering chemicals;
2. development of a comfortable, drug-free lifestyle;
3. an understanding of the process of addiction and recovery;
4. establishment and maintainance of a program which supports lasting recovery.

Although the cocaine recovery support groups operate in a context that offers a continuum of care, including long-term residential treatment and short-term crisis detoxification, the groups described in this chapter are conducted on an outpatient basis. This mode, however, can also be applied with some modification in a residential setting. While attending outpatient group sessions, clients are strongly encouraged to participate concurrently in Alcoholics Anonymous, Narcotics Anonymous, Cocaine Anonymous, and other self-help programs which support a chemical-free lifestyle and promote emotional, social, and spiritual growth. The cocaine recovery support group may be the only treatment for some, but most clients use it in combination or in sequence with the other modalities. We do not encourage the client to think of the group as the entire course of treatment, but to view it as part of a full program of recovery. Members of the client's family are also involved in the treatment process through family sessions, couple's sessions, or Al-Anon and Nar-Anon meetings.

The core of our treatment approach is the peer group, composed of similar people voluntarily seeking solutions to similar problems. The group interacts through care, support, and honest and immediate confrontation among members. The group setting provides an opportunity to identify with peers in a way which mitigates the feelings of uniqueness, guilt, and shame which many clients bring to treatment. Cocaine-specific groups allow this identification to happen readily, and also offer ample opportunity to provide useful education to clients regarding the psychological and physiological effects of the drug. We had initially hypothesized that drug-related paranoia and/or an inflated regard for social status might preclude a group therapy approach, especially with high-dose cocaine users. Our experience, however, indicates group treatment actually relieves anxiety and helps clients overcome feelings of isolation and omniscience. In cases where actual toxic psychosis exists we refer the client to residential detoxification until their acute symptoms have abated.

THE LANGUAGE OF RECOVERY

Our cocaine recovery support groups have primarily utilized traditional concepts of recovery from addiction. The direction of the groups is derived from the model and principles of recovery outlined in the Twelve Steps and Traditions of Alcoholics Anonymous, Narcotics Anonymous, and Cocaine Anonymous. One of the major goals of the cocaine recovery groups is to provide a bridge to A.A., N.A., and C.A.; not only to bring about an awareness of these resources, but to demonstrate the ways in which they are essential to recovery.

A basic theme and focus in the group is learning and internalizing the language and the process of recovery, as exemplified by A.A. This language is precise, but foreign to most people. It is an epistemology which creates a new system of values and beliefs and a new way of looking at the world and learning about oneself, one's relationships to others, and the addictive process.

The initial task of the cocaine group is to help the client replace common generalized notions of willpower or impulse control with internalized, specific concepts of recovery that have personal meaning. For example, by thinking in terms of a force of will, one is led to feelings of guilt and self-recrimination for past failures. By replacing willpower with an acceptance of powerlessness over the drug, the client is able to shift from the destructive guilt process — feeling weak, bad, crazy, and stupid — to the constructive process of taking responsible action in recovery. Clearly defined changes in the client's attitude and behavior are the eventual goal. When a client has accepted powerlessness, often he or she will be less likely to resort to denial, be more willing to ask for help, and be more ready to incorporate that help in recovery. The basis of this reframing process is similar to that which underlies the Twelve Steps of Alcoholics Anonymous.[2,3,4]

The process is also eloquently described by Gregory Bateson in his 1971 paper, "Cybernetics of Self: A Theory of

Alcoholism."[5] Bateson's major contention is that the use of willpower to control or stop addictive drinking is not only counterproductive, but dangerous and often fatal. The alcoholic/addict and society generally are preoccupied with the myth of self-control: "If I only had more willpower, I could. . .," "If he only had more strength. . .," etc. Bateson describes his attempts at working with alcoholics and admits failure when applying psychotherapeutic techniques. He then describes his gratitude to some of his patients who had introduced him to Alcoholics Anonymous and the language of recovery. Within the First Step of the A.A. program lies the key which unlocks the addictive trap. With the admission of powerlessness over alcohol, cocaine, and other drugs, one gains power over the rest of one's life.

A metaphor that illustrates the paradoxical nature of this experience is a description of the children's toy called the Chinese finger puzzle. The puzzle is a small, tubular basket in which one inserts the index fingers of both hands. As any child will discover after some experimenting, the harder one pulls to get free, the tighter the basket becomes. In order to extricate oneself from the trap, it is necessary to give up, relax, and push slightly in the opposite direction. In order to begin recovery from addiction, the same is true: willpower and controlled use are ideas which actually prolong the struggle and entrapment.

Within the language of recovery there are three distinct experiences:

- ADMISSION
- ACCEPTANCE
- SURRENDER

The first step in the process of recovery is admitting the addiction exists. When people enter the group they often verbally and intellectually admit they have a problem with cocaine. While this admission is an essential beginning, it is usually inadequate for maintaining a lasting recovery. The group sessions help people move from this intellectual admission to an experiential acceptance of their inability to control drug use. As is the case with alcoholic clients, denial and other defenses are not easily dismantled. Often we will challenge the more difficult clients to attempt controlling or limiting their cocaine use in some manner. When they fail, their full acceptance of that fact marks the beginning of the recovery process. These experiences are then shared and examined in the group. This particular technique would not be useful in a residential setting, where commitment to abstinence is a prerequisite for admission to treatment. In the outpatient groups, however, it is sometimes part of the process of making a commitment to abstinence. Repeated failure to achieve control or abstinence often leads the client to recognize the need for residential treatment and to accept a referral previously refused.

While the experience of acceptance is difficult to convey in words, it is apparent in actual behavioral changes. Acceptance of addiction opens up the possibility of making a commitment to abstinence which is not just verbal, but leads to noticeable changes in the client's lifestyle. For example, many initiate steady attendance at N.A., C.A., and A.A. meetings and begin to develop support systems comprised of people who do not use cocaine or other drugs.

Surrender is a much deeper level of acceptance where the struggle with the addiction ceases, and the person actively and positively decides to give up all the enervating and usually unsuccessful efforts at controlled use. Surrender is the difference between willing something to happen and becoming willing for something to happen. One gives up, lets go of the need to control drug use, and becomes willing to accept help. Dr. Harry M. Tiebout describes this experience as follows:

> We can now be more precise in our definition of an act of surrender. It is to be viewed as a moment when the unconscious forces of defiance and grandiosity actually cease

effectively to function. When that happens, the individual is wide open to reality; he can listen and learn without conflict and fighting back. He is receptive to life, not antagonistic. He senses a feeling of relatedness and an at-oneness which become the sources of an inner peace and serenity, the possession of which frees the individual from his compulsion to use. In other words, an act of surrender is an occasion when the individual no longer fights life but accepts it.

Having defined an act of surrender as a moment of accepting reality on the unconscious level, it is now possible to define the emotional state of surrender as one in which there is a persisting capacity to accept reality. In this definition the capacity to accept reality must not be conceived of in a passive sense but in the active sense of reality being a place where one can live and function as a person acknowledging one's responsibilities and feeling free to make that reality more livable for oneself and others. There is no sense of 'must' nor is there any sense of fatalism. When true unconscious surrender has occurred the acceptance of reality means that the individual can work in it and with it. The state of surrender is really positive and creative.[6]

PHASES OF TREATMENT

The treatment process can be divided roughly into three phases, each involving specific tasks and emphases:
1. establishing abstinence and sobriety;
2. developing a comfortable, drug-free lifestyle;
3. dealing with issues of arrested maturity and delayed withdrawal.

Movement through these phases of treatment is not necessarily in sequence. The groups are designed to include individuals who are in various stages of treatment and recovery.

Thus, clients who are working on establishing abstinence are in group with others who have been drug free for a year or more. Just as social pressure is one of the motivations for drug use, peer group pressure can motivate recovery as well as support it. People whose recovery is well established lend credibility to what is taught in the groups by sharing their experience. Those in early stages of recovery help to counteract the selective memory (euphoric recall) of cocaine use which often emerges after a period of abstinence.

Establishing Abstinence and Sobriety

One of the primary tasks in establishing abstinence is to help clients recognize and accept that they have, and will continue to have, the urge to use cocaine. Rather than repress or deny this urge, we encourage them to accept the fact that they are having the experience, and to talk about it with the group and with others who are part of a support system identified for this purpose. One of the frequently repeated maxims in the group is a quote from David E. Smith, "Silence is the enemy of recovery."[7] This applies especially to the experience of drug hunger.

In addition to talking about the conscious and specific urge to use cocaine, we work on identifying the more subtle feeling states and environmental triggers which often precede the craving for cocaine. For example, many clients report the following environmental stimuli as triggers for cocaine hunger: substantial amounts of cash, familiar pieces of music, sexual arousal, driving by the dealer's house, seeing people and places associated with cocaine use, drug paraphernalia, and the use of other drugs. For most people, the most powerful environmental trigger seems to be physical proximity to the drug.

Drug hunger can also be triggered by a variety of internal stimuli. These are usually identified in retrospect by examining patterns of experience and tracing them back to the earliest warning signs; for example, feelings of boredom, loneliness, or lethargy. With this focus and practice in the group sessions, people gradually become skilled in recognizing the urge in its nascent forms, when it is easier to take alternative or preventive action. The client can then begin to allow drug hunger to trigger alternative activities.

Part of the first treatment phase is the development of action plans for avoiding situations and experiences which trigger drug hunger. Another ingredient in this phase is education. We teach that the urge to use exists in a primary and primitive part of the brain and is energized by both a powerful biochemical process and a strongly conditioned learning history. Explaining the pharmacology of cocaine in simple language is often a very liberating factor in early recovery because the client is absolved of blame for having the urge. The important point now, however, is that the client needs to learn how to take responsibility for developing alternative behaviors when the urge arises. The urge to use is automatic, but by consistent practice, one can develop other healthful responses.

Specific suggestions for alternatives to drug use in early recovery include frequent attendance at A.A., N.A., or C.A. meetings, regular aerobic exercise (which aids in physical detoxification), slow, long distance running, deep relaxation techniques, acupuncture, and biofeedback. A balanced diet is also helpful for maintaining recovery. These activities can help speed up the process of detoxification and the restoration of the body's natural biochemical balance, which happens over an extended period of time. They are also useful in management of anxiety, stress, and "empty time," and provide a sense of purpose and confidence. While research has been published in some of these areas, it is beyond the scope of this chapter to discuss specific mechanisms.[8]

We also teach that once an individual develops addictive disease and the compulsion to use is established, it remains intact for life. However, once abstinence is achieved and the urge to use is no longer acted on, drug hunger diminishes in frequency and intensity. Resumption of use at any stage of recovery reconstitutes the compulsion at its highest level of intensity. Thus, there is no possibility of returning to controlled use, and recovery becomes a life-long process of learning to live comfortably and responsibly without the use of any psychoactive substance.

One of the critical factors in establishing abstinence is understanding the danger in using drugs other than cocaine. In addition to the obvious danger of substitution, other psychoactive chemicals (alcohol and marijuana being the most common) tend both to activate the compulsion and to lower the resistance to use cocaine. This has been the experience of the vast majority of our clients, and may be due to a combination of biochemical and environmental factors. The encouragement of total drug abstinence provides the widest margin of safety and avoids the dangers of possible substitution or relapse. We take the issue of relapse very seriously, as any relapse could be fatal.

Developing a Comfortable, Drug-Free Lifestyle

Once abstinence has been achieved, we encourage people to take the steps necessary to maintain it and to live a comfortable, self-fulfilling life in recovery. The major task of the second stage of treatment is to confront the problems created by the addiction and to deepen and expand the commitment to a drug-free lifestyle. This involves more than simply abstaining from drugs. Group members support each other to assess aspects of their behavior and patterns in their relationships which are a source of pain for themselves and those around them. We explore ways of making amends for negative behavior which occurred during the active phases of addiction and work on establishing positive alternatives to the old patterns. This is similar to the Ninth Step of Alcoholics Anonymous. Just as it is important to acknowledge the reality of one's past, it is equally critical to develop the ability to let go of the guilt and resentment which past actions have engendered. If this is not accomplished, recovery is likely to be undermined and relapse becomes possible. The techniques we use in group to accomplish these ends can be characterized as reality-oriented, cognitive, behavioral therapy.[9]

In addition to our group work, we also encourage members to deal with these issues through the relationships they have developed in A.A., N.A., and C.A. fellowships. We believe attendance in the cocaine recovery group once a week does not provide sufficient attention and energy sufficient for making the necessary changes. We recommend group members design a program which includes a minimum of three activities per week which directly address their recovery. We monitor and discuss this in group sessions by having each client check in and describe to the group their recovery-oriented activities of the previous week.

Once abstinence is firmly established, feelings are more readily accessed without the danger of causing relapse and without the retreat into the confusion and disassociation which often accompany active drug use. In the second phase of treatment, group discussion is not limited to drug-related behavior, but includes other aspects of experience. The language of recovery is as integral to this phase as it is to the establishment of abstinence. Here relationship and sexual issues are prominent and more easily focused on. The group provides not only an opportunity to share common experiences, but an actual arena in which to access old patterns and practice new ways of relating to others.

Learning to recognize and accept the entire breadth of one's feelings is essential to the recovery process. In order to begin to practice this acceptance, it is necessary to understand the difference between "sitting on" (repression/avoidance/denial) and "sitting with" feelings (acceptance/surrender). We actually illustrate and practice the awareness of this difference in group. The new perception becomes a tool which members use in their daily lives. The outcome of this particular practice is the willingness to take responsibility for one's feelings, rather than continuing the old patterns of guilt, blame, and resentment. As Stephen Levine said:

> Many are encouraged to "take responsibility" for their illness but are seldom taught the difference between responsibility and blame. Many, when taking responsibility for their illness but finding themselves unable to change its course, feel guilty for not being responsible. But responsibility is not blame; it is the ability to respond, which comes out of being present in the moment.[10]

Dealing with Delayed Withdrawal and Arrested Maturity

While recovery is a lifelong process of growth, treatment is a time-limited experience. The particular rhythm and duration of treatment varies from individual to individual, but we generally recommend that clients remain active in treatment for twelve to eighteen months. The rationale for this is twofold. First, our experience with recovering cocaine addicts indicates there are definite flare-up periods, similar to those which have been well documented in recovery from alcoholism. Although there appears to be little clinical research on this phenomenon, it seems to involve a delayed withdrawal syndrome, characterized by a reemergence of many of the classical symptoms associated with early withdrawal such as anxiety, depression, irritability, sleep disturbance, and compulsiveness with food (especially sugars). This complex of symptoms can occur following a stressful situation, but it often frustratingly occurs out of the blue, without any identifiable external or internal stressors. In either case, the risk of relapse is intensified, and it is useful for the client to be active in the group when these periods occur. Actually, these flare-up periods tend to occur with some predictability at around the third month, between the ninth and twelfth month, and occasionally as late as the eighteenth month following abstinence.

In group sessions, we help clients recognize this syndrome and understand the experience as part of the healing process in recovery. The sharing of information and experience about the universality of this phenomenon helps counteract feelings of discouragement or panic which tend to accompany it. During flare-up periods, we encourage clients to intensify their use of resources for support and nurturing, and we take time in the group to help them develop specific strategies in this regard. As in all phases of treatment, we work towards helping them verbalize and accept their feelings and to respond in new and more constructive ways. We also encourage them to attend more A.A., N.A., or C.A. meetings where the response to their experiences is often "you're right on schedule."

Another issue in the final phase of treatment, which generally begins after about a year of recovery, is the problem of arrested maturity.[11] During the progression of chemical dependency, regardless of age at onset, drug use becomes the primary means of responding to emotional and interpersonal issues. Alternative responses fail to develop beyond this point. The development of self-awareness, self-esteem, and the capacity for real intimacy with others is severely curtailed; the earlier the onset of addiction, the greater the deficits. Once drug use has ceased, a realistic program for maintaining recovery has been established, and the immediate aspects of "clearing up the wreckage" have been accomplished, the recovering person is ready to resume personal growth by addressing repressed feelings and unresolved conflicts. The goals and techniques employed here are like those of traditional therapies, with the addition of a constant sensitivity and attention to the specific issues of recovery.

Another predominant task in the later stage of treatment is developing the spiritual dimension of one's life. This is the key element in lasting recovery, and a substantial amount of group time is spent helping people discover and develop a spiritual practice in their lives. The nature of this practice is not easily generalized because it is so intensely personal. Some examples of spiritual tools we encourage clients to use in recovery are daily meditation, prayer, and reflective reading. One purpose of these practices is to counteract the tendency to become obsessed with negative thoughts and expectations and to mitigate anxiety and stress. More importantly, spiritual practices help build self-confidence and faith in a Power greater than oneself. This faith in turn becomes a powerful antidote to fear.

SUMMARY

We have attempted to make clear that the recovery process is life-long. In its early phases, clients are working primarily to achieve relief from guilt and pain created by their addiction. As recovery progresses, however, there is a movement from a feeling of relief to a true experience of delight.[12] The goals of treatment have been achieved when this shift is evident, when one is living comfortably, responsibly, and joyfully without cocaine or other drugs.

Our experience indicates that treating cocaine addicts in cocaine-specific groups is useful in that the homogeneity facilitates group identification and the educational component of treatment. However, the content of the groups and the nature of the recovery process are not drug-specific or unique. The emergence of Cocaine Anonymous, which is based upon the same Twelve Steps as Alcoholics Anonymous, also illustrates this. What we are treating is addictive disease, not alcoholism, cocaine addiction, etc. Regardless of the chemical, the essentials of treatment are the same; the language of recovery is universal.

The authors wish to express heartfelt appreciation to Millicent Buxton, Dr. Joseph McCarthy, and Dr. David E. Smith for their work as cofacilitators in the cocaine recovery support groups and their help in developing the models described in this chapter. We also wish to thank Lawrence Ross and Michael Sparks for their invaluable editorial advice.

Chapter 5
ENDNOTES

1. R. K. Siegal, "Cocaine Smoking." *Journal of Psychoactive Drugs,* Vol. 14, No. 4, 1982.
2. *Alcoholics Anonymous.* (New York: A.A. World Services, Inc., 1976). Available through Hazelden Educational Materials, order no. 2020.
3. *Twelve Steps and Twelve Traditions.* (New York: A.A. World Services, Inc., 1980). Available through Hazelden Educational Materials, order no. 2080.
4. E. Kurtz, *Not-God: A History of Alcoholics Anonymous.* (Center City, MN: Hazelden Educational Materials, 1979). Order no. 1036.
5. G. Bateson, *Steps to An Ecology of Mind.* (New York: Ballentine, 1975).
6. H. M. Tiebout, "The Act of Surrender in the Therapeutic Process." *Quarterly Journal of Studies on Alcoholism,* 10:48-59. Available through Hazelden Educational Materials, order no. 4360.
7. D. E. Smith, "Diagnostic, Treatment, and Aftercare Approaches to Cocaine Abuse." *Journal of Substance Abuse Treatment,* Vol. 1, No. 1, pp. 5-9, 1984.
8. R. E. Seymour and D. E. Smith, *Alternatives to Alcohol and Drug Abuse.* (New York: Sarah Lazin Books, in press).
9. W. Glasser, *Reality Therapy: A New Approach to Psychiatry.* (New York: Harper & Row, 1965). Available through Hazelden Educational Materials, order no. 6605.
10. S. Levine, *Who Dies? (An Investigation of Conscious Living and Conscious Dying).* (Garden City, NY: Doubleday Anchor Books, 1982).

11. J. Milam, *Under the Influence: A Guide to the Myths and Realities of Alcoholism.* (Seattle, WA: Madrone Publishers, Inc., 1981).
12. J. Enright, *Enlightening Gestalt.* (Mill Valley, CA: Pro Telos, 1980).

BIBLIOGRAPHY

Cohen, S. *Cocaine Today.* (Rockville, MD: American Council on Marijuana and Other Psychoactive Drugs, 1981).

Hampden-Turner, C. *Maps of the Mind.* (New York: MacMillan Publishing Co., Inc., 1981).

Phillips, J., and Wynne, R. *Cocaine.* (New York: Avon Books, 1980).

Smith, D. E., and Wesson, D. R., "Cocaine." *Journal of Psychedelic Drugs,* Vol. 10, No. 4, Oct.-Dec., 1978.

Smith, D. E., et. al. "Treatment Considerations with Cocaine Abusers." *Cocaine: A Second Look,* (Rockville, MD: American Council on Marijuana and Other Psychoactive Drugs, 1983).

Appendix
UPDATE ON COCAINE DEPENDENCE: CRACK AND ADVANCES IN DIAGNOSTICS AND TREATMENT
Mim Landry

Over the past few years more and more people have been using central nervous system stimulants in general and cocaine in particular. Of special interest is the increased use of *rapid-delivery* forms of stimulants, with the best example being *crack or rock cocaine* which is smoked rather than snorted. This general increase in the use of stimulants, coupled with a rise in the use of rapid delivery systems, has increased the possibility and probability of acute toxic reactions and the development of addiction to cocaine and other psychoactive drugs.

Over these same past few years significant clinical advances have been made in the diagnosis and treatment of addictive disorders. Recent revisions to the Psychoactive Substance Use Disorders section of the American Psychiatric Association's *Diagnostic and Statistical Manual of Mental Disorders (DSM-III-R)* provide the clinician with an effective diagnostic tool to identify early psychoactive drug dependence.

Of equal importance are advances made in the understanding of the neurochemistry and subsequent pharmacological treatment of addictive disorders, particularly with cocaine dependence. Such advances include the use of amino acid neurotransmitter precursor loading for depleted neurotransmitters; the use of dopamine receptor agonists such as bromocriptine or amantadine, which simulate postsynaptic receptor actions of depleted neurotransmitterrs; and even the use of tricyclic antidepressants which can increase the amount of existing neurotransmitters in the synapse.[1,2,3,4]

This appendix will provide comprehensive understanding of the more recent changes and advances in cocaine and crack use and research. It will also provide the health care professional with additional tools necessary to treat the cocaine-dependent person.

WHAT IS COCAINE AND CRACK COCAINE?

Cocaine is an alkaloid prepared from the Erythroxylum coca plant. Cocaine hydrochloride (HCL) is prepared by dissolving the alkaloid in hydrochloric acid to form a water-soluble salt. This decomposes with heat, has a melting point of 195 degrees centigrade, and is called *cocaine HCL*.

Because cocaine HCL vaporizes at a fairly high temperature, much of it is destroyed if it is smoked. It is usually snorted intranasally or injected. Until recently most cocaine bought, sold, and used in the United States was in the form of cocaine hydrochloride.

Cocaine HCL can also be changed back into the alkaloidal state with a free-basing kit. This is commonly called free-base cocaine or "crack." Free-base cocaine is formed when the cocaine alkaloid is freed from its hydrochloride salt. This cocaine melts at low temperatures and vaporizes at slightly higher temperatures. It is not destroyed by heating and thus is easily smoked or, more accurately, as the cocaine melts and vaporizes, the cocaine "smoker" inhales the vapors.

Cocaine used in this free-based state is ideal for achieving the drug euphoria sought by users. Inhaled cocaine vapors are absorbed directly into the lungs. The pulmonary route provides rapid transport of cocaine from the lungs into the user's brain; the process takes seven seconds. After snorting cocaine, it takes 30 to 120 minutes for levels in the plasma to rise significantly.[5] The rise is also far less significant than with inhaled cocaine vapors. The chart labeled "Single Use of Cocaine—Effect on Emotions" describes the role that route of administration plays in understanding cocaine

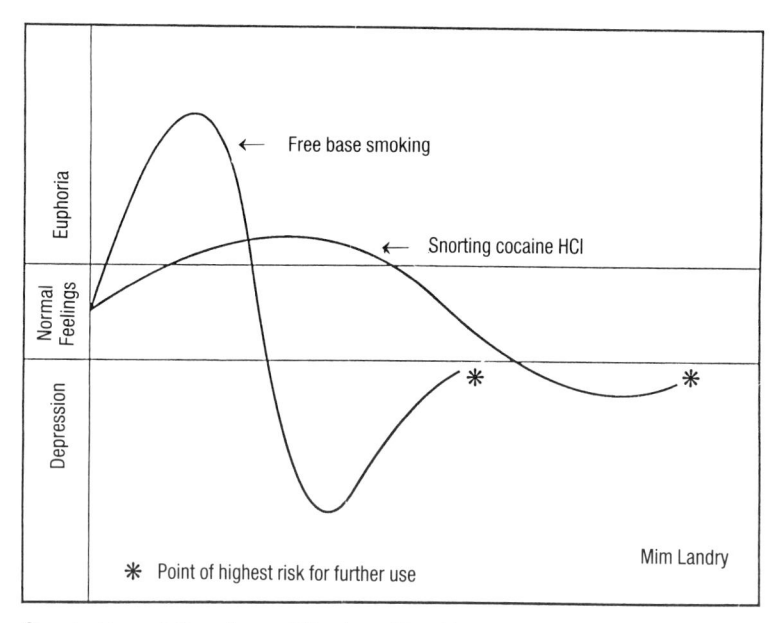

Single Use of Cocaine - Effect on Emotions

Chart labels: Euphoria / Normal Feelings / Depression; Free base smoking; Snorting cocaine HCl; ✶ Point of highest risk for further use; Mim Landry

euphoria and other psychological effects. The rapid rise of cocaine levels in the plasma via smoking yields a significant euphoria, but also ushers in a dramatic and marked depression following the euphoria.

Classic free-base methods involve kits using ether or other chemicals which are messy and often highly inflammable. Crack cocaine is popular because cocaine HCL can be inexpensively and easily processed with baking soda and water, yielding a ready-to-smoke form of free-base cocaine. Crack could not have been marketed any better. It is sold in small, inexpensive units, smoked in glass pipes, or just sprinkled on tobacco or marijuana. Thus, cocaine in a smokable form is available at a cost of five to twenty dollars.

Euphoria from cocaine smoking is as intense as it is short. Because plasma saturation of cocaine is high via the pulmonary route, the cocaine smoker gets very high, very quickly. It is felt that the immediate euphoria is the result of a surge in neurotransmitters, including serotonin, dopamine, and norepinephrine. During acute cocaine use, elevated mood is the result of an acute increase of neurotransmitters. However, a dopamine depletion hypothesis, discussed later in this appendix, helps to explain the resultant depression that follows cocaine euphoria.[6]

COMPULSION TO USE DRUGS

Compulsive drug use can develop in various ways. For example, someone who has tolerance to and dependence on heroin or alcohol may use those drugs for their primary effect as well as to avoid withdrawal symptoms. Psychoactive drugs may produce positive reinforcement, promoting continued drug-taking behavior. Drug use patterns and the negative consequences of drug use may also reinforce continued drug taking.

Cocaine has a very pronounced positive reinforcement value. Its effect upon the central nervous system (CNS) provides remarkably positive reinforcement, especially if smoked. In contrast, the depression that follows cocaine euphoria is notoriously negative. Therefore, cocaine users are motivated to smoke additional cocaine to self-medicate the depression. This helps to initiate and sustain compulsive, addictive cocaine dependency.

Considering the positive reinforcement properties of cocaine, the tendency to self-medicate cocaine-induced negative states, and the resultant cocaine-induced euphoria-depression cycle, the following five items characterize cocaine smoking:

1. The development of compulsion is rapid.

2. The compulsion to use and especially to smoke cocaine is very powerful.

3. The user tends to use increasingly higher doses of cocaine and will typically progress to more effective and dangerous delivery systems.

4. The user will self-medicate the stimulant side-effects with a CNS depressant, and tend to use increasingly higher doses of the CNS depressant.

5. The tendency toward higher doses of cocaine and CNS depressants, more effective delivery systems, and increased time using the drugs puts the user at a higher risk for experiencing toxic effects of cocaine (and other drugs) and development of addiction.[7]

It appears that food and water reward the human brain via the dopaminergic system. Similarly, cocaine's ability to satiate the user's need for food, sex, and sleep may be a function of its known dopaminergic activity, along with other mechanisms. Even though it may be discovered that the mechanisms are different, it is likely that cocaine shares a common anatomical link with natural, positive reinforcers like food and sex.

DIAGNOSTIC UPDATE

Health care professionals in all specialty areas may encounter patients who have psychoactive substance use disorders. But because of a wide variety of reasons, they may not accurately identify, diagnose, and treat the disorder. Until recently, few medical, nursing, or social work schools, or psychology or psychiatric departments, taught accurate, up-to-date information about the treatment of addictive disease. More attention has been paid to the consequences of addiction rather than to the diagnoses and treatment of addictive disease. For example, all medical schools will teach the treatment of medical pathology secondary to alcoholism, but few have addressed the actual treatment of alcoholism itself. For this and other reasons, there has long been much controversy regarding the nature of addiction, as well as how to identify and treat it.

One area of concern has been the philosophical foundation upon which treatment strategies rest. For example, traditional psychology and psychiatry have held that substance use disorders are typically the result of some other psychiatric problem. The treatment goals would be to treat the underlying psychopathology in the hopes that the drug abuse problems would disappear. Another view, commonly called the *disease concept of addiction,* holds that addiction is a primary disorder and needs to be treated as such.[8] In this regard, there has been confusion as to the difference between addiction to legal drugs versus illicit drugs. For example, alcohol is a legal and, for the most part, socially acceptable drug (although often not considered to be a drug per se), while marijuana, heroin, and cocaine are unacceptable in most sectors of society. These culturally and societally influenced views have little to do with the psychopharmacology and neurochemistry of substance abuse, but do lead to significant and critical misunderstandings about the process of addiction.

To counteract this, the American Medical Association passed a resolution stating that addictions to all psychoactive drugs are to be understood as diseases. The resolution concludes as follows:

> Resolved that the American Medical Association endorses the proposition that drug dependencies, including alcoholism, are diseases, and that their treatment is a legitimate part of medical practice; and that the AMA encourages individual physicians and other health professionals, medical and other health-related organizations, and governments and other policy-makers to become more well-informed about drug dependencies, to base their policies and activities on recognitions of drug dependency.[9]

If it can be understood that a disease is a pathological process with characteristic signs and symptoms, then a reliable diagnosis should describe most people who have that disease. A disease should also have a predictable prognosis, or theory about how the pathology will proceed if left untreated or unchecked. Intervention in the pathological process is a form of treatment that aims to reduce or eliminate this process. Beyond this, there should be a way to provide tools for living beyond the acute treatment stage—that is, there should be a recovery process.

Addictionology, the medical specialty for the study and treatment of addictive disorders, has stressed that drug abuse is the use of a psychoactive drug interfering with a person's physical, psychological, emotional, social, occupational, spiritual, or financial life. Addiction is best seen as a pathological process that is progressive and life-threatening if left untreated. The characteristic signs and symptoms of the addictive process are (1) compulsion to use a psychoactive drug, (2) loss of control over the use of a psychoactive drug, (3) continued use of a psychoactive drug despite adverse consequences, and (4) a strong potential for the return to the use of a drug after treatment (relapse).[10, 11] Note that these descriptions do *not* rely on the specific pharmacology of the drug in question, as was the case with the previous reliance on the presence of a withdrawal syndrome of the alcohol type.

In the past, the presence of a withdrawal syndrome along with social or occupational impairment were the two chief symptoms used to describe addiction.[12] The reliance on physical tolerance and dependence as well as social or occupational impairment was faulty for two primary reasons. First, both of these processes are often *late stage* problems. Second, the pharmacology of drugs differs, making reliance on pharmacological processes such as tolerance and withdrawal a poor choice.[13] Recognizing this, the *DSM-III-R* deviates significantly from past editions.

COCAINE DEPENDENCE

The *DSM-III-R* describes nine symptoms for cocaine dependence, noting that three or more are necessary to fulfill the diagnostic criteria:

1. substance often taken in larger amounts or over a longer period than the person intended

2. persistent desire or one or more unsuccessful efforts to cut down or control substance use

3. a great deal of time spent in activities necessary to get the substance (e.g., theft), taking the substance (e.g., chain-smoking), or recovering from its effects

4. frequent intoxication or withdrawal symptoms when expected to fulfill major role obligations at work, school, or home (e.g., does not go to work because hung over, goes to school or work "high," intoxicated while taking care of his or her children), or when substance use is physically hazardous (e.g., drives when intoxicated)

5. important social, occupational, or recreational activities given up or reduced because of substance use

6. continued substance use despite knowledge of having a persistent or recurrent social, psychological, or physical problem that is caused or exacerbated by the use of the substance (e.g., family arguments about it, cocaine-induced depression, or having an ulcer made worse by drinking)

7. marked tolerance: need for markedly increased amounts of the substance (i.e., at least a 50 percent increase) in order to achieve intoxication or desired effect, or markedly diminished effect with continued use of the same amount

8. characteristic withdrawal symptoms of depression, agitation, anxiety, lethargy, dysphoria

9. substance often taken to relieve or avoid withdrawal symptoms[14]*

In addition to requiring at least three of the above criterion to arrive at a diagnosis of cocaine dependence, some symptoms of the disturbance should have persisted for at least one month, or have occurred repeatedly over a longer period of time, according to the *DSM-III-R*.

It is critical to note that use of the word *dependence* in the phrase cocaine dependence in *DSM-III-R* very clearly denotes a process of addiction that may or may not refer to physical dependence. Dependence here means *addiction* or the commonly used phrase *chemical dependency.*

Note that the criterion deal with loss of control (1 and 2), time involvement (3), social dysfunction (4 and 5), continued use despite adverse consequences (6), development of tolerance and withdrawal (7, 8, and 9).

---

*All references to the *Diagnostic and Statistical Manual for Mental Disorders, Third Edition, Revised* are reprinted with permission from the *Diagnostic and Statistical Manual for Mental Disorders, Third Edition, Revised*, Copyright 1987, American Psychiatric Association.

Determining Severity of Dependence

The *DSM-III-R* also describes criteria for the *severity* of cocaine dependence:

Mild: Few, if any symptoms in excess of those required to make the diagnosis, and the symptoms result in no more than mild impairment in occupational functioning or in usual social activities or relationships with others.

Moderate: Symptoms or functional impairment between "mild" and "severe."

Severe: Many symptoms in excess of those required to make the diagnosis, and the symptoms markedly interfere with occupational functioning or with usual social activities or relationships with others.

In Partial Remission: During the past six months, some use of the substance and some symptoms of dependence.

In Full Remission: During the past six months, either no use of the substance, or use of the substance and no symptoms of dependence.[15]

The inclusion of the severity index is both useful and problematic. As a description of human behavior, the severity of addiction is a legitimate issue and an important clinical concept. However, the description of *mild* cocaine dependence is precariously close to the diagnostic criteria for cocaine *abuse.*

COCAINE ABUSE

The *DSM-III-R* describes the diagnostic criteria for cocaine *abuse* as follows:

A. A maladaptive pattern of cocaine use indicated by at least one of the following:
   (1) continued use despite knowledge of having a persistent or recurrent social, occupational, psychological, or physical problem that is caused or exacerbated by use of the psychoactive substance

  (2) recurrent use in situations in which use is physically hazardous (e.g., driving while intoxicated)
B. Some symptoms of the disturbance have persisted for at least one month, or have occurred repeatedly over a longer period of time.
C. Never met the criteria for [cocaine dependence.][16]

 In short, abuse is described as drug use that creates some type of dysfunction, or drug use that potentially could create a significant problem. The *DSM-III-R* describes abuse and dependence categories for alcohol, sedative-hypnotic-anxiolytics, opioids, cocaine, amphetamines, PCP, hallucinogens, cannabis, inhalants, and nicotine dependence. The *DSM-III-R* also describes two residual abuse and dependence categories for drugs that cannot be classified according to the previous categories or for use in situations where the specific substance is not yet known. There is also a classification for polysubstance dependence, where a person has repeatedly used at least three categories of psychoactive substances, but where no single drug predominates.

COCAINE-INDUCED ORGANIC MENTAL DISORDERS

 In addition to describing cocaine dependence and cocaine abuse, the *DSM-III-R* also describes four additional cocaine-related problems: cocaine intoxication, cocaine withdrawal, cocaine delirium, and cocaine delusional disorder.

Cocaine Intoxication

 Cocaine intoxication is the acute, or short-term response to a potent central nervous system stimulant. Physical symptoms include increased motor activity and blood pressure, psychomotor agitation, tachycardia, loquacity or speech compression, and possible perspiration and chills. Psychological symptoms may include antidepression or even the characteristic cocaine euphoria, grandiosity, and feelings of well-being, power, and control. There may be a heightened sexual interest or perhaps sexual interest and behavior that is normally repugnant to the individual in a sober state. As an example, a conservative, married man may engage in homosexual sex only during active cocaine use. More severe symptoms may include hypervigilance, grandiosity, and repetitive, stereotypical, perversive behavior. The *DSM-III-R* diagnostic criteria for *cocaine intoxication* includes:

   A. Recent use of cocaine.
   B. Maladaptive behavior changes, e.g., euphoria, fighting, grandiosity, hypervigilance, psychomotor agitation, impaired judgment, impaired social or occupational functioning.
   C. At least two of the following signs appear within one hour of using cocaine:
      1. tachycardia
      2. pupillary dilation
      3. elevated blood pressure
      4. perspiration or chills
      5. nausea or vomiting
      6. visual or tactile hallucination
   D. Not due to any physical or other mental disorder.[17]

The chart on page 93, titled, "Single Use of Cocaine—Effect on Emotions," describes the initial response to a single dose of cocaine. The chart compares the difference between snorting cocaine hydrochloride and smoking cocaine in the free base state, such as crack cocaine. Clearly, the pulmonary route of administration provides for more intense symptoms, as does the amount of cocaine used, the purity of the cocaine, and other variables such as total drug combinations and sleep and food deprivation.

Cocaine Crash

As the "Single Use of Cocaine" chart shows, the cocaine euphoria is quickly followed by a marked depression. These rebound effects are primarily dysphoric in nature and are typically accompanied by intense cocaine hunger. While depression and fatigue are typical features, stimulant effects including nervousness, irritability, and anxiety will remain. This is perhaps the most serious trigger point for the return to cocaine use.

Cocaine Withdrawal

Should the cocaine crash persist beyond twenty-four hours, the *DSM-III-R* notes that the crash should be termed "cocaine withdrawal." Cocaine withdrawal is noted for the marked depressive, dysphoric mood of the client. There is often irritability, anxiety, fatigue, and insomnia. There may also be severe depression and suicidal thoughts; some chronic users, especially those who have taken higher doses, may also feel paranoia. The cocaine withdrawal typically peaks within one to four days, although irritability and depression may linger for a few months.

The *DSM-III-R* criteria for *cocaine withdrawal* is as follows:
A. Cessation of prolonged heavy use of cocaine or a reduction in the amount of cocaine used, followed by dysphoric mood (e.g., depression, irritability, and anxiety) and at least one of the following, persisting more than 24 hours after cessation of substance use:
   1. fatigue
   2. insomnia or hypersomnia
   3. psychomotor agitation
B. Not due to any physical or other mental disorder.[18]

Cocaine Psychosis and Delirium

One of the more troubling problems related to cocaine use is the potential for a cocaine-induced delirium. This is characterized by poor attention to external stimuli, inability to shift attention to new external stimuli, disorganized thinking, sensory misperceptions, and disorientation as to time, place, and person. Importantly, violence, and aggressive and belligerent behavior is common, and the person may engage in maladaptable behavior. The delirium typically occurs within an hour of medium- or high-dose cocaine use and may last a few hours.

The *DSM-III-R* describes *cocaine delirium* as follows:
A. Reduced ability to maintain attention to external stimuli and to appropriately shift attention to new external stimuli.
B. Disorganized thinking, as indicated by rambling, irrelevant, or incoherent speech.
C. At least two of the following:
   1. reduced level of consciousness
   2. perceptual disturbances: misinterpretations, illusions, or hallucinations
   3. disturbance of sleep-wake cycle with insomnia or daytime sleepiness
   4. increased or decreased psychomotor activity
   5. disorientation to time, place, or person
   6. memory impairment, e.g., inability to learn new material or remember past events such as history
D. Clinical features develop over a short period of time.
E. Delirium developing within 24 hours of use of cocaine.
F. Not due to any physical or other mental disorder.[19]

Cocaine Delusional Disorder

Cocaine, like other stimulants (and other drugs), can create a delusional syndrome with typical feelings of persecution, often shortly after initiation of drug use. It may begin as distortions and misperceptions, such as of body image. Suspiciousness and curiosity may be replaced by persecutory delusions and violent actions based on those delusions. There may also be the presence of formications, or "coke bugs," which are tactile hallucinations of bugs crawling on or under the skin, resulting in picking at the imaginary bugs, producing numerous skin sores.

The *DSM-III-R* describes *cocaine delusional disorder* as follows:
A. Organic Delusional Syndrome developing shortly after the use of cocaine.
B. Rapidly developing persecutory delusions are the predominant clinical feature.
C. Not due to any physical or other mental disorder.[20]

MEDICAL MANAGEMENT OF COCAINE OVERDOSE

For cocaine intoxication, diazepam 10 mg PO may be given for anxiety, paranoia, and hyperexcitability. An appropriate psychiatric consultation should be made if symptoms escalate. Also there should be a referral to an addictionologist or a chemical dependency treatment program.

For more critical CNS stimulation problems such as hallucinations, extreme paranoia, and destructive behaviors, hospital admission is recommended. Adequate precautions should be taken relative to suicidal and homicidal activities. For sedation and anticonvulsant prophylasis, consider diazepam 5 mg IV q five minutes for a maximum of four doses; or amobarbital 20-75 mg IV q five minutes for a maximum of four doses. Attempts at sedating patients with neuroleptics such as haloperidol or chlorpromazine in the acute cocaine overdose stage are dangerous, for these drugs lower seizure threshold. Some seizures are refractory to diazepam, and for these, consider thiopental 50-100 mg IV and succinylcholine 40-100 mg IV. This will stop seizures and will facilitate intubation. These procedures should only be performed by a physician trained in emergency medicine and with a life-support system available.

Following intubation, provide mechanical ventilation by ambu bag or a volume respirator, with FiO_2 titrated to arterial blood gases. Respiratory alkalosis tends to resolve as the patient's respirations slow. Also, start cardiac monitoring and check vital signs frequently to detect ventricular arrythmias and hypertension.

G.R. Gay has developed the following system for the treatment of persistent adrenergic crisis:
1. Carefully monitor signs of CNS, cardiovascular system and respiratory system in timed sequence.
2. Administer propranolol either:
   (a) in slow intravenous increments of 1 mg at one minute intervals, up to a total of 6 mg; or
   (b) orally, in doses of 40-80 mg at four to six hour intervals

for a period of up to one week, titrated by radial pulse rate (a pulse of 90 or less is the goal).
3. Give sips of 5 percent glucose solution, possibly cranberry juice rich in benzoid acid.
4. Acidify urine with intravenous ammonium chloride (NH4C1), at 75 mg/kg, QID (maximum dosage 6 gr per day).
5. Apply the "Science of Art" (described below).
6. As an adjunctive therapy, administer diazepam at bedtime. This propranalol protocol will reverse the hyperkinetic state within three to five minutes after intravenous administration and within 20-40 minutes with oral administration.[21, 22]

The "Science of Art"

Gay's "Science of Art" reminds physicians that a patient is in a psychological as well as dopaminergic crisis. The acronym ART reminds us to provide nonpunitive, nonjudgmental, humane care.

"A" stands for *acceptance*. Acceptance lends credibility. Caring intermediaries help cocaine users adapt to and regulate their environment as drug effects dissipate.

"R" stands for *reduction* of stimuli, rest, and reassurance. A quiet, nonthreatening environment and a gentle (yet professional) approach generates gratitude and greatly diminishes anxiety and potential for destructive behaviors.

"T" stands for *talk down* technique. Verbal sincerity, concern, and a gentle manipulation of the patient's psyche are particularly important to the cocaine user. Users may misinterpret insincere or abrupt actions as being hostile. Initially, talk down is best carried out in a designated calm place with individualized counseling, massage of muscle spasms, and mild sedation.[23]

It is critical to remember that the management of cocaine-related medical pathology is not treatment for cocaine dependence.

For some cocaine users, medical management of the acute cocaine withdrawal state is basically stopping cocaine and other drug use, establishing proper nutrition and aerobic exercise habits, resuming normal sleep patterns, and learning about cocaine addiction.

Other clients, particularly chronic or high-dose cocaine users and those who have been involved in a polydrug use pattern, may experience more profound symptoms. These may include depression, agitation, irritability, anergia, and cocaine hunger. Clients with preexisting psychiatric problems may experience symptom reemergence, which will complicate the detoxification and recovery process.

Detoxification for Polydrug Addicts

For the polydrug addict, particularly the cocaine-alcohol addict, tolerance to alcohol may determine the direction of the detoxification process. If dependence on alcohol exists (especially if it is significant), the withdrawal symptoms from alcohol may overshadow those of cocaine. Therefore, detoxification from alcohol becomes the primary goal and can be treated in a standard fashion.

The cocaine-benzodiazepine addict may have symptoms similar to alcohol withdrawal, though possibly for a longer time. Some of these clients may experience a three-week period of significant agitation, anxiety, and insomnia. However, if a benzodiazepine dependency syndrome is suspected, it may be necessary to focus on the benzodiazepine dependency. Smith and Wesson have described a phenobarbitol substitution technique for benzodiazepine dependency.[24] If symptoms are detoxification-related they will fade over time. If they represent a return of underlying symptomatology, the symptoms will increase in severity.

After detoxification, the goal is to have the patient establish and maintain sobriety from all psychoactive drugs. Natural peptides, such as the beta-endorphins and enkaphalins, play an important role in combating drug hunger and creating a sense of well-being. Regular aerobic exercise such as running or swimming increases available endorphins. Aerobic exercise three times per week helps to restore endorphin levels and assists the person to handle stress, anxiety, and pain.

UPDATE ON NEUROCHEMISTRY AND COCAINE

Cocaine, like all psychoactive drugs, affects and alters brain chemistry (or neurochemistry) significantly. Although our knowledge of cocaine-related neurochemistry is in its infancy, a growing body of knowledge can provide the health care professional with understanding of cocaine-induced effects and rationales for pharmacological treatment.[25, 26] Existing studies have generally focused on cocaine's effect on the dopamine, norepinephrine, and serotonin neurological pathways.

Dopamine, norepinephrine, and serotonin are neurochemicals called *neurotransmitters* that are responsible for the smooth functioning of nerve signal transmission and mental health. Because neurons are physically separated from each other, nerve impulses must "jump" from neuron A to neuron B at the gap between the neurons called the *synaptic gap* or *synapse*. These impulses are suppressed or stimulated through a number of mechanisms, including the status of the neurochemistry of the synapse. Cocaine affects these neurotransmitters acutely and chronically. As a generalization, with the initial administration of cocaine, these neurotransmitters tend to increase in number, leading to increased nerve impulses within that pathway. However, with chronic use of cocaine, these neurotransmitters are generally depleted, decreasing nerve impulses within that pathway. It is necessary to briefly describe these three pathways to understand both the action of cocaine on the body as well as to understand treatment rationales.

Cocaine's Effect on the Dopamine System

The dopaminergic system is related to smooth motor control, and to the limbic system that is responsible for the regulation of emotional behavior.[27] Cocaine affects the normal operation of this neurological pathway by blocking the reuptake of dopamine, stimulating dopamine release. Normally, dopamine released in the synaptic cleft of a dopaminergic neuron will, after stimulating the post-synaptic neuron, reenter the presynaptic neuron through a process called reuptake.

Cocaine blocks this reuptake process and therefore leaves more dopamine in the synapse, creating a "flood" of dopamine. This dopaminergic flood creates the well-known cocaine euphoria. However, with chronic use of cocaine, and the continued blockage of the reuptake system and resulting decrease in the recycling of dopamine, the net outcome is dopamine depletion. Evidence suggests that the dopamine system reacts to a chronic depletion of dopamine by dopamine receptor supersensitivity—that is, increased numbers of dopamine receptor sites.[28]

Cocaine's Effect on the Norepinephrine System

Cocaine's effect on the norepinephrine or adrenergic system is related to cocaine-related central and peripheral nervous system stimulation symptoms. These include increases in pulse, blood pressure, tremor, dilated pupils, and other classic stimulant symptoms such as increased motor activity and agitation. Cocaine blocks the reuptake of norepinephrine as well as facilitating norepinephrine release centrally and peripherally. It is thought that cocaine also activates norepinephrine inhibitory presynaptic autoreceptors. Chronic exposure to cocaine will increase norepinephrine pre- and post-synpatic receptor density, resulting in increased sensitivity following chronic cocaine use.

Cocaine's Effect on the Serotonin System

Serotonin is the neurotransmitter related to a sense of well-being, mood, sleep, aggression, and arousal. It appears that cocaine affects serotonin by blocking the uptake of tryptophan, the amino acid precursor to serotonin. With chronic use of cocaine, it is likely that there is a decrease in serotonin synthesis and metabolism.

Chronic serotonin depletion may cause serotonin receptors to become supersensitive, and these receptors may be responsible for some of the cocaine withdrawal symptoms.

PHARMACOLOGICAL TREATMENT OF COCAINE WITHDRAWAL

Amino Acids

Cocaine reduces the available stores of serotonin, dopamine, and norepinephrine. These depletions of neurotransmitters either create or are important in the cocaine withdrawal syndrome. Also, cocaine is an effective appetite suppressant, further reducing the intake of amino acids necessary for smooth neurochemical functioning. Therefore, the use of tyrosine or DL Phenylalanine (the amino acid precursors to dopamine and norepinephrine) and L-tryptophan (the amino acid precursor to serotonin) is a rational choice for reestablishing neurochemical homeostasis.

Wesson and Smith are studying the role of L-tryptophan in cocaine withdrawal treatment, hypothesizing that serotonin receptors may experience supersensitivity or upregulation as a result of serotonin depletion.[29] The use of L-tryptophan may replenish the available stores of serotonin, and promote the downregulation of serotonin receptors, reducing cocaine withdrawal symptoms. While controlled studies of individual amino acids are necessary for scholarly and treatment advances, Tennant[30] and Rosen and Flemenbaum[31] recommend the combination of tyrosine and levodopa, both precursors to dopamine and norepinephrine. Gold and others[32,33,34] used L-tyrosine as treatment for cocaine withdrawal symptoms, and studies report that depression, irritability, and anxiety were reduced in their cocaine patients. Others recommend using a combination of tyrosine and tryptophan. Trachtenberg and Blum have developed a product for cocaine withdrawal which combines tyrosine, tryptophan D- and L-Phenylalanine, glutamine, along with vitamins and minerals.[35] Controlled studies are under way. Table 1 provides a rationale for the combined use of tyrosine and L-tryptophan.

TABLE 1

PHARMACOLOGICAL TREATMENT OF COCAINE WITHDRAWAL

Amino Acids:
 tyrosine 400 mg TID, X 1-4 weeks
 L-tryptophan 1500 mg hs X 1-4 weeks
 Note: Give tyrosine between meals, on an empty stomach; Give L-tryptophan with high carbohydrate diet.

Amantadine: 100 mg bid-qid x 4 weeks
 Note: Caution regarding seizure and psychosis. Precursor loading with tyrosine is expected and recommended.

Desipramine: 250 mg hs X 8 weeks
 Note: Start at 50 mg and increase.

Bromocriptine: 0.625 mg to 2.5 mg TID-QID x 4 weeks
 Note: Stress importance of lower dosage: sensitivity and side-effects.

Amantadine

Amantadine hydrochloride is a medication prescribed for treatment of Parkinson's disease and an antiviral agent for treatment of Influenza-A. Amantadine also promotes the release of dopamine from dopaminergic neurons and slows the reuptake of dopamine. The net result of amantadine intake is increased dopamine availability in the synaptic cleft. However, amantadine may also create dopamine depletion, so Tennant and Sagherian recommend that amantadine be taken in combination with tyrosine and levodopa.[36]

Table 1 describes a rationale for amantadine use for cocaine withdrawal.

Desipramine

The use of tricyclic antidepressants is compelling but controversial in that it is likely that only a minority of cocaine addicts have genuine endogenous depression. Because a chief feature of cocaine withdrawal for chronic cocaine users is depression, which may last from a few weeks to a few months, the use of antidepressants may be a rational pharmacological alternative. However, Gawin and Kleber note that desipramine decreases cocaine craving after two to three weeks of treatment.[37] This is supported by Rosecan, who points to the efficacy of using desipramine for cocaine craving and depression.[38] However, despramine, like many other tricyclics, needs approximately two weeks to take effect.

Bromocriptine

Bromocriptine is a dopamine receptor agonist which activates postsynaptic dopamine receptors directly. Like amantadine, bromocriptine is used to treat the symptoms of Parkinson's disease and affects the dopaminergic system. Whereas amantadine causes the release of dopamine from the presynaptic neuron (and slows dopamine reuptake), bromocriptine basically "tricks" the postsynaptic neuron into thinking that it is dopamine and causes neuronal firing. Dackis et al. noted that bromocriptine administration resulted in cocaine craving.[39] They also warned about using neuroleptics such as thioridazine, which may provoke cocaine craving. Tennant and Sagherian have also utilized bromocriptine and noted sensitivity problems such as headaches.[40] Others who have seen benefits from the use of bromocriptine for cocaine withdrawal include Giannini et al.[41], Dackis and Gold[42], Sweeney, Byronhs, and Climko[43], and Pottash.[44] Table 1 provides a model for use.

SUMMARY

Increased use of cocaine and the recent introduction of crack cocaine has propelled the medical establishment to make significant advances in the understanding of the diagnosis and treatment of addictive disease. First, crack provided an excellent model for understanding how the same drug—cocaine—could create an amazingly wide variety of effects, depending on the route of administration (snorted versus smoked). Second, crack has helped diagnosticians to realize that addictive disease is often unrelated to simple pharmacological actions such as tolerance and tissue dependence. Third, crack has spurred research into the neurochemical foundations of cocaine dependence, and hence spawned various theoretical and pragmatic lines of pharmacological treatment for cocaine dependence.

As we enter the 1990s there will be continued discoveries related to the diagnosis and treatment of addictive disease. There may be important research findings related to biological markers for addiction, which will become standard tools for addiction professionals. Similarly, advances in neurochemical research may develop pharmacological "cures" for addictive behavior.

It is important that these tools always remain within the context of a multidisciplinary team approach to the treatment of chemical dependency, recognizing the continuum of care. Pharmacological treatment of chemical dependency must always be understood as one of many available tools which include the Twelve Step programs of Cocaine Anonymous, Alcoholics Anonymous, Narcotics Anonymous, alcoholism/drug abuse counselors, nurse specialists in chemical dependency, addictionologists, other physicians, and pharmacists. Advances in chemical dependency treatment should best support and augment, but not replace, the multidisciplinary approaches to the treatment of addictive disease.

APPENDIX
ENDNOTES

1. M. S. Gold, A. L. Pottash, W. J. Annito, K. Verebey, and D. R. Sweeney, "Cocaine Withdrawal: Efficacy of Tyrosine," *Neurosic Abstract*, 9 (1983): 157.
2. K. Blum, M. C. Trachtenberg, "Neurochemistry and Alcohol Craving," *California Society for the Treatment of Alcoholism and Other Drug Dependencies News*, 13 (1986): 1-7.
3. F. S. Tennant, Jr., A. A. Sagherian, "Double-Blind Comparison of Amantadine and Bromocriptine for Ambulatory Withdrawal from Cocaine Dependence," *Archives of Internal Medicine*, 147 (1987): 109-12.
4. Robert D. Doigle, H. Westley Clark, and M. J. Landry, "A Primer on Neurotransmitters and Cocaine," *Journal of Psychoactive Drugs*, 20 (1988): 3.
5. T. Tommasello, "Cocaine Dependence and Treatment: The Pharmacological Aspects," *PharmAlert*, 15 (Fall 1984): 1-3.
6. C. A. Dackis, M. S. Gold, R. K. Davis, and D. R. Sweeney, "Bromocriptine Treatment for Cocaine Abuse: The Dopamine Depletion Hypothesis," *International Journal of Psychiatry in Medicine*, (1985).
7. M. J. Landry, D. E. Smith, "Crack: Anatomy of an Addiction," *California Nursing Review*, 9 (1987): 2.
8. D. E. Smith, H. B. Milkman, and S. G. Sunderwirth, "Addictive Disease: Concepts and Controversy," *The Addictions: Multidisciplinary Perspectives and Treatments* (Lexington, Mass.: Lexington Books, 1985), 145-60.
9. A. Meacham, "AMA Declares All Drug Dependencies Diseases," *The U.S. Journal of Drug and Alcohol Dependence*, 11 (1987): 1-2.
10. Smith, Milkman, and Sunderwirth, "Addictive Disease: Concepts and Controversy," *The Addictions: Multidisciplinary Perspectives and Treatments* (Lexington, Mass.: Lexington Books, 1985), 145-60.

11. D. E. Smith and M. J. Landry, "Psychoactive Substance Use Disorders: Drugs and Alcohol," H. H. Goldman ed., *Review of General Psychiatry* (Los Altos, Calif.: Lange Medical Publications, 1988).
12. American Psychiatric Association, *Diagnostic and Statistical Manual of Mental Disorders, Third Edition, Revised* (Washington, D.C.: American Psychiatric Association, 1987).
13. M. J. Landry, "Addiction Diagnostic Update: (DSM-III-R) Psychoactive Substance Use Disorders," *Journal of Psychoactive Drugs*, 19 (1987): 4.
14. American Psychiatric Association, *DSM-III-R*, 167-168.
15. Ibid., 168.
16. Ibid., 169.
17. Ibid., 142.
18. Ibid., 142-143
19. Ibid., 143-144
20. Ibid., 144
21. G. R. Gay, "You've Come a Long Way, Baby! Coke Time for the New American Lady of the Eighties," *Journal of Psychoactive Drugs*, 13 (1981): 297-317.
22. G. R. Gay, D. S. Inaba, W. Sheppard, and J. A. Newmeyer, "Cocaine: History, Epidemiology, Human Pharmacology and Treatment," *Clinical Toxicology*, 8 (1975): 2.
23. Gay, "You've Come a Long Way, Baby!" 297-317.
24. D. E. Smith and D. R. Wesson, "Benzodiazepine Dependency Syndromes," *Journal of Psychoactive Drugs*, 15 (1983): 1-2.
25. A. M. Washton and M. S. Gold, *Cocaine: A Clinician's Handbook* (New York: The Guildford Press, 1987).
26. T. Tommasello, "Cocaine Dependence and Treatment: The Pharmacological Aspects," *PharmAlert*, 15 (Fall 1984): 1-3.
27. C. A. Dackis and M. S. Gold, "Pharmacological Approaches to Cocaine Addiction," *Journal of Substance Abuse Treatment*, 2 (1985): 3.
28. F. S. Tennant, "Effect of Cocaine Dependence on Plasma Phenylalanine and Tyrosine Levels and on Urinary MHPG

Excretion," *American Journal of Psychiatry*, 142 (1985): 1200-1201.
29. D. R. Wesson and D. E. Smith, conversation with author: Ongoing research at the Meritt Peralta Institute Chemical Dependency Recovery Hospital, Oakland, California.
30. F. S. Tennant, "Effect of Cocaine Dependence on Plasma Phenylalanine and Tyrosine Levels and on Urinary MHPG Excretion," *American Journal of Psychiatry*, 142 (1985): 1200-1201.
31. H. Rosen, A. Flemenbaum, and V. Slater, "Clinical Trial of Carbidopa-L-Dopa Combinations for Cocaine Abuse," *American Journal of Psychiatry*, 143 (1986): 11.
32. M. S. Gold, A. L. Pottash, W. J. Annitto, K. Vereby, and D. R. Sweeney, "Cocaine Withdrawal: Efficacy of Tyrosine." Paper presented at the thirteenth annual meeting of the Society for Neuroscience, Boston, Nov. 6-11, 1983.
33. C. A. Dackis and M. S. Gold, "New Concepts in Cocaine Addiction: The Dopamine Depletion Hypothesis," *Neuroscience and Biobehavioral Reviews*, 9 (1985).
34. M. S. Gold, A. M. Washton, and C. A. Dackis, "Cocaine Abuse: Neurochemistry, Phenomenology and Treatment," *NIDA Research Monograph* No. 61, (1985).
35. M. C. Trachtenberg and K. Blum, "Cocaine and Neurochemical Functioning: The Use of Tropamine in Treatment, Relapse Prevention and the Recovery Process." Matrix Technologies, Houston, Texas.
36. Tennant and Sagherian, "Double-Blind Comparison."
37. F. H. Gawin and H. D. Kleber, "Cocaine Abuse Treatment. Open Pilot Trial with Desipramine and Lithium Carbonate," *Archives of General Psychiatry*, 41 (Sept. 1984).
38. J. S. Rosecan and E. V. Nunes, "Pharmacological Management of Cocaine Abuse," H. I. Spitz and J. S. Rosecan, eds., *Cocaine Abuse: New Directions in Treatment and Research* (New York: Brunner/Mazel, 1987).
39. C. A. Dackis, M. S. Gold, R. K. Davis, and D. R. Sweeney, "Bromocriptine Treatment for Cocaine Abuse: The Dopamine

Depletion Hypothesis," *International Journal of Psychiatry in Medicine*, 15 (1986): 2.
40. Tennant and Sagherian, "Double-Blind Comparison."
41. A. J. Giannini, P. Baumgartel, and L. R. DiMarzio, "Bromocriptine Therapy in Cocaine Withdrawal," *Journal of Clinical Pharmacology*, 27 (1987): 4.
42. C. A. Dackis and M. S. Gold, "Pharmacological Approaches to Cocaine Addiction," *Journal of Substance Abuse Treatment*, 2 (1985): 139-45.
43. C. A. Dackis, M. S. Gold, D. R. Sweeney, U. P. Byronhs, and R. Climko, "Single Dose Bromocriptine Reverses Cocaine Craving," *Psychiatry Research*, 29 (April 1987).
44. C. A. Dackis, M. S. Gold, and A. L. Pottash, "Central Stimulant Abuse: Neurochemistry and Pharmacology" (New York: Haworth Press, 1987).

Other titles that will interest you...

Ethics for Addiction Professionals
by LeClair Bissell, M.D., C.A.C., and James E. Royce, S.J., Ph.D.

This book leads the discussion about the crucial and complex ethical issues facing professionals in the addiction field today. Timely and thought-provoking, it points out the necessity of standard guidelines for professional conduct by raising several key questions about confidentiality, mandatory reporting, personal relationships and more. 60 pp.
Order No. 5028

Cocaine
Beyond the Looking Glass
A Hazelden Film by Dick Young

Suitable for adolescents, families, church and community groups, as well as chemically dependent people, this award-winning film provides timely information from recovering addicts about the experience of cocaine addiction—and the hope available through Narcotics Anonymous. Available in 16mm, ½" VHS, and ¾" video formats. 28 minutes

The Physiological Effects of Cocaine
A Hazelden Educational Materials Production

A discussion for professionals of cocaine's effect upon bodily systems. The film includes physiological and psychiatric toxicology information to help counselors respond to cocaine addicts in treatment. Viewers' notes are included. Available in ½" VHS and ¾" video formats. 20 minutes

To order, or for information about purchasing or renting films, please call one of our Customer Service Representatives.

HAZELDEN EDUCATIONAL MATERIALS

(800) 328-9000	**(800) 257-0070**	**(612) 257-4010**
(Toll Free. U.S. Only)	(Toll Free. MN Only)	(AK and Outside U.S.)

Pleasant Valley Road • Box 176 • Center City, MN 55012-0176